BIRTH, SUFFERING AND DEATH

Philosophy and Medicine 41

BIRTH, SUFFERING, AND DEATH

CATHOLIC PERSPECTIVES
AT THE EDGES OF LIFE

Edited by

KEVIN Wm. WILDES, S.J.

Center for Ethics, Medicine and Public Issues,
Baylor College of Medicine, Houston, Texas, U.S.A.

FRANCESC ABEL, S.J.

Institut Borja de Bioetica, Barcelona, Spain

JOHN C. HARVEY

Centre for Clinical Bioethics, Georgetown University, Washington, D.C., U.S.A.

KLUWER ACADEMIC PUBLISHERS
DORDRECHT / BOSTON / LONDON

Library of Congress Cataloging-in-Publication Data

Birth, suffering, and death : Catholic perspectives at the edges of
  life / edited by Kevin Wm. Wildes, Francesc Abel, John C. Harvey.
      p.   cm. -- (Philosophy and medicine ; v. 41) (Catholic
  studies in bioethics)
    Includes index.
    ISBN 0-7923-1547-2 (alk. paper)
    1. Life and death, Power over--Religious aspects--Catholic Church.
  2. Medical ethics. 3. Bioethics. 4. Christian ethics--Catholic
  authors. 5. Catholic Church--Doctrines.   I. Wildes, Kevin Wm.
  (Kevin William), 1954-   . II. Abel, Francesc. III. Harvey, John
  Collins. IV. Series. V. Series: Catholic studies in bioethics.
  BJ1469.B57 1992
  241'.6424--dc20   91-40540

ISBN 0-7923-1547-2

Published by Kluwer Academic Publishers,
P.O. Box 17, 3300 AA Dordrecht, The Netherlands.

Kluwer Academic Publishers incorporates
the publishing programmes of
D. Reidel, Martinus Nijhoff, Dr W. Junk and MTP Press.

Sold and distributed in the U.S.A. and Canada
by Kluwer Academic Publishers Group,
101 Philip Drive, Norwell, MA 02061, U.S.A.

In all other countries, sold and distributed
by Kluwer Academic Publishers,
P.O. Box 322, 3300 AH Dordrecht, The Netherlands.

printed on acid-free paper

Printed in the Netherlands

TABLE OF CONTENTS

ACKNOWLEDGEMENTS

Tables 1, 2, 3, and 4, in *The HIV Infection,* are from R. H. Rubin, "Acquired immunodeficiency syndrome", in *Scientific American Medicine, E. Rubenstein (ed.), 1989, Annals of Internal Medicine.*

Figure 1, in *"The HIV Infection* is an illustration in AIDS 1988", by R. C. Gallo and L. Montagnier, in *Scientific American,* October 1988, p. 43.

Figure 2, *in The HIV Infection,* is an illustration in "The Moleclar Biology of the AIDS Virus", by W. A. Haseltine and F. Wong-Staal, in *Scientific American,* October 1988, p. 51.

Figure 3, in *The HIV Infection,* is an illustration, by Ian Worpole, in "HIV Infection: The Clinical Picture," by R. Redfield and D. Burke, in *Scientific American,* October 1988, p. 97.

Figure 4 in *The HIV Infection,* is an illustration by Ian Worpole, in "HIV Infection: The Clinical Picture," by R. Redfield and D. Burke, in *Scientific American,* October 1988, p. 94.

Figure 5 in *The HIV Infection* is an illustration, by Hank Iken, in "AIDS Therapies," by R. Yarchoan, H. Mitsuya, and S. Broder, in *Scientific American,* October 1988, p. 112.

"Declaration on Euthanasia," reprinted with permission of The United States Catholic Conference.

"The Prolongation of Life", reprinted with permission of *The Pope Speaks,* 1958, Vol. 4, pp. 393–398.

EDMUND D. PELLEGRINO

FOREWORD

For centuries the Roman Catholic Church has been concerned with the moral implications of medical practice. Indeed, until two decades ago, Catholic moral theologians were the major source of moral guidance, scholarly reflection and teaching on a variety of medical-moral topics, particularly those bearing on human life. Many, not only those within the Catholic communion, turned to the Church for guidance as each new possibility for altering the conditions of human life posed new challenges to long held moral values.

Two decades ago, the center of gravity of ethical reflection shifted sharply from theologians and Christian philosophers to more secular thinkers. A confluence of forces was responsible for this metamorphosis – an exponential rate of increase in medical technologies, expanded education of the public, the growth of participatory democracy, the entry of courts and legislation into what had previously been private matters, the trend of morality towards pluralism and individual freedom and the depreciation of church and religious doctrines generally. Most significant was the entry of professional philosophers into the debate, for the first time. It is a curious paradox that, until the mid-sixties, professional philosophers largely ignored medical ethics. Today they are the most influential shapers of public and professional opinion.

As a result, the character of contemporary biomedical ethical discourse has become predominantly secular. Subjects of the utmost importance – abortion, euthanasia, assisted suicide, terminating life support, surrogate parenthood, definitions of death, personhood, and individuality, the ontological status of the embryo, to name a few, are all treated in ways which prescind from, and even depreciate, religious values. Contemporary philosophical ethics is predominantly pluralistic, libertarian, and individualistic. It is antipathetic to natural law arguments. Its ethos is relativistic, strongly utilitarian and inclined to social, cultural and historical determinism. In this intellectual climate religious arguments are inadmissable. To cope with the loss of metaphysical foundations, procedural ethics has virtually displaced substantive ethics. Many deny

ix

K.Wm. Wildes (ed.), Birth, Suffering and Death, ix–x.
© 1992 Kluwer Academic Publishers. Printed in the Netherlands.

that there is any "foundation" for bioethics except autonomy, or coherence and "consensus" among and between, competing ethical theories. In this context religious commitments are considered outmoded, "unreasonable" and divisive. Any source of moral authority other than law or public consensus is discredited. Believers whatever their persuasion are virtually disenfranchised in public policy debates.

Given the profoundly non-theological orientation of biomedical ethics today there is urgent need for a more visible, witness to the Catholic Perspective on Medical Morals. To be effective that witness must be informed, intelligent, and scholarly. It must be in dialogue with the mainstream of thinkers in secular biomedical ethics. The Christian ethical points of view must be authentically, responsibly, and charitably presented. Such an effort must be international and trans-cultural, since medical progress presents a world-wide challenge to moral values.

The new series inaugurated with this volume, is a welcome addition to the expanding world literature in biomedical ethics. It offers a forum in which qualified scholars in the Roman Catholic Tradition may present their critical reflections for Catholics and non-Catholics alike. This series will complement the Philosophy and Medicine series also published by Kluwer. Edited as it is by a panel of international scholars, the new series promises to reach a wide audience among theologians, health professionals, and moral philosophers.

To the Editors: Ad multos Annos!

FRANCESC ABEL S.J. AND JOHN C. HARVEY

PREFACE

Pope John XXIII said at the opening of the Second Vatican Council: "Recent research and discoveries in the sciences, in history, and in philosophy bring up new problems which have an important bearing on life itself and demand new scrutiny by theologians" (Pope John XXIII). The late Dr. André Hellegers, the founder of the Kennedy Institute of Ethics at Georgetown University, in 1972 echoed Pope John's words. He insisted that there was a real need for careful, serious, and prayerful dialogue between biomedical scientists and medical practitioners on the one hand and Roman Catholic philosophers and theologians on the other. He recognized that the magnificent new and unprecedented advances in medical science and technology had brought concomitant problems concerning moral behavior which added even greater urgency for such dialogues. New and correct scientific facts need to be incorporated into the reflections of ethicists and moral theologians so that in light of newly discovered knowledge a keener discernment of the Revelation may be possible. Accurate knowledge or truth is always presupposed in moral affirmations about human behavior. And truth may be found, Thomas asserted, on the basis of human reason reflecting on human nature in the light of faith.

Pope John Paul II addressed the issue of ethics and medicine on October 27, 1980. When speaking in an audience granted to the members of the Italian Society of Internal Medicine and the Italian Society of General Surgery, on the occasion of their annual meeting held in Rome, the Pope appealed to the physicians to help in promoting a science that is tailored to man's real needs and not a science merely pursuing technological progress and organizational efficiency for its own sake (Pope John Paul II). As a response to this appeal of the Holy Father, in March of 1981 representatives of some member universities of the International Federation of Catholic Universities (IFCU) and other institutions met in Milan under the Chairmanship of the Rector Magnificus of the Catholic University of Italy, Professor Giuseppe Lazzati, to organize a group that could promote the type of dialogue referred to above. In time the group

xi

K.Wm. Wildes (ed.), Birth, Suffering and Death, xi–xv.
© 1992 *Kluwer Academic Publishers. Printed in the Netherlands.*

was organized as the International Study Group on Bioethics (ISGB) of the IFCU.

The main goal of the ISGB is to promote dialogue among medical scientists on the one hand and Roman Catholic ethicists and moral theologians on the other. As a first step this dialogue was limited to Roman Catholic ethicists and moral theologians, but as time goes on it is to be expanded into an ecumenical dialogue. By this means it is hoped that the ethicists and theologians will have correct and timely facts concerning whatever biomedical and technological advances they may discuss. Thus they may incorporate into their ethical reflections the most up-to-date scientific knowledge. Such exchanges of information, with the subsequent identification of the moral problems which arise, may enhance the exploration of the solutions to these identified moral problems. The ISGB has from the beginning of its work offered the fruits of these dialogues to the Magisterium from loyal members of the Church.

Since 1981, some 19 dialogues have been held. Invited participants have included prominent and knowledgeable biomedical scientists and medical practitioners, of various religious persuasions and each a noted figure in his or her field, and Roman Catholic philosophers and theologians reflecting both conservative and liberal views. Some of the subjects covered in these dialogues have been: the concept of nature; embryology; growth and development; genetic engineering; human genetics and neonatology; foetal therapeutics; genetic treatment; new obstetrical technologies; definitions of death; the persistent vegetative state; and modern epidemic diseases.

To insure free, open, and uninhibited discussion of these subjects from the scientific and ethical viewpoints, it was determined at the outset that no record of the proceedings would be published. Individual participants found that the dialogues have been rich, fruitful, and illuminating. It has always been the policy that individual participants were free to publish their own presentation if they so wished. Many of the individual participants have subsequently published a reworking of their paper in one or another scholarly journal (e.g., Demmer, 1988). The ISGB came to the realization that much valuable philosophical and theological reflection upon these topics was being lost. In 1988 it collected some of the articles already published individually and republished them, with permission, as a collection concerned issues surrounding the beginnings of life (Abel, Boné, Harvey, 1988).

It became apparent from this endeavor that a vehicle was needed to offer those scholars who participated in the dialogues and who wished to do so, the opportunity of publishing their reflections in a timely manner and as a part of a group of essays organized about a particular biomedical topic or technology. Such an opportunity came about when the editors and publisher of the series *Philosophy and Medicine* conceived the idea of a subseries for Catholic bioethics. Thus the series *Catholic Studies in Bioethics* was born!

Initially one volume will be published annually. The series will have only an indirect relation to the ISGB. It will have editors and an editorial board independent of the ISGB and responsible only to the editors of the series *Philosophy and Medicine* and the publisher. It will, however, give preference to any participant in any of the dialogues sponsored by the ISGB for consideration of publication of his or her paper. Other papers fitting the topic under discussion will be solicited from appropriate scholars as required for completeness in the exploration of a given topic.

Both the Editors are members of the ISGB. The Associate Editor is the managing editor for the *Journal of Philosophy and Medicine*. The Editors, Associate Editor, and all members of the Editorial Board as well, are active practicing Catholic scholars in one or more fields of medicine, biomedical science, ministry, ethics, or moral theology. They are an international group. They represent a cross-generational age mix. They come from diverse educational and cultural backgrounds. They represent varying viewpoints from conservative to liberal within the Roman Catholic tradition. A listing of these individuals and their qualifications follows:

Name	Degree	Institution Awarding	Field	Current Position
Francesc Abel, S.J.	D.Med. M.A. S.T.L.	University of Barcelona	Med. (GYN), Ethics, Demography Moral Theology	Director, Borja Institute of Bioethics, Barcelona
Antonio Autiero	D.Phil. D.Theol.	Pontifical Latern University	Moral Theology	Prof. of Theology, University of Münster
Thomas J. Bole, III	Ph.D.	University of Texas	Moral Theology	Prof. Med. Ethics University of Oklahoma, U.S.A.
Paolo Catorini	D.Med. D.Phil.	U. of Pavia Catholic U. of Italy	Philosophy of Medicine Medical Ethics	Coord., School of Med. Hum., Institute San Raffaele, Milan

Klaus Demmer	S. T. D.	Pontifical Gregorian University	Moral Theology	Professor of Moral Theology, Pontifical Gregorian University
Josef F. Fuchs S.J.	D. Theol.	University of Münster	Moral Theology	Professor of Moral Theology, Emeritus, Potifical Gregorian University
Erny Gillen	S.T.D.	Catholic University of Louvain	Moral Theology	Secretary General, Caritatas, Luxemburg
John Collins Harvey	M.D. Ph.D.	Johns Hopkins St. Mary's U. (Baltimore)	Med. (Geriatrics), Bioethics, Moral Theology	Prof. Med. Emeritus, Georgetown U., Sen. Research Scholar, Kennedy Institute
John M. Haas	S.T.L Ph.D.	University of Fribourg Catholic University of America	Moral Theology	Professor of Moral Thelogy, St. Charles Borromeo Seminary
Bernard Hoose	S.T.D.	Pontifical Gregorian University	Moral Theology	Lecturer, Missionary Institute, London
Johannes Huber	D. Med. D. Theol.	University of Vienna	Med. (OB/GYN), Mor. Theol.	Assoc. Prof. of OB/GYN, Univ. of Vienna
William M. Joensen	M.A. (Theol.)	Pontifical Coll. Jospehinum (Ohio)	Pastoral Ministry, Mor. Theol.	Associate Pastor, Sacred Heart Church, Waterloo, Iowa, USA
James F. Keenan, S.J.	S.T.D.	Pontifical Gregorian University	Moral Theology	Asst. Prof. Theol., Weston School of Theology, Cambridge, Mass.
James J. McCartney, OSA	Ph.D.	Georgetown University	Moral Theology	Assoc. Prof. Phil., Villanova U., Penn.
Jean Porter	Ph.D.	Yale University	Christ. Eth., Mor. Theol.	Asst. Prof. U. of Notre Dame, Indiana
Frank H. Rossi	S.T.L.	Pontifical lateran University	Pastoral Ministry, Mor. Theol.	Vice-Chancellor, Diocese of Galveston-Houston, Texas
Edward C. Vacek, S.J.	Ph.D.	Northwestern University	Mor. Theol., Pastoral Theology	Assoc. Prof. Weston School of Theol., Cambridge, Mass.

Paul J.M. van Tongeren	Ph.D.	Catholic University of Louvain	Moral Philosophy	Prof. Moral Phil., Cath. U. Nijmegen
Matthias Volkenandt	D.Med. Dipl. Theol.	University of Bonn	Med. (Oncology), Moral Theology	Fellow, Sloan-Kettering Cancer Center, New York
James J. Walter	Ph.D.	Catholic University of Louvain	Christ. Eth., Mor. Theol.	Prof. Christ. Eth., Loyola U., Chicago
Kevin W. Wildes, S.J.	M.S. M.Div. M.A. M.A.	Fordham Weston Weston Rice U.	Philos. Ministry Theology Philosophy	Center for Ethics, Medicine & Public Issues, Baylor College of Medicine, Houston, Texas

Each volume will deal with a particular topic relating to medical discovery, praxis, or technology which creates ethical problems needful of consideration. The contents of that volume will explore that topic form the scientific, ethical, social, and theological considerations within the context of the Roman Catholic tradition. In no sense will these essays be the final words on such subjects – that is the task of the authoritative Magisterium. These presentations will merely be the reflections of the invited scholars contributing their thoughts upon the topics in the hopes of furthering our understanding of a solution to these human problems. In this way the dialogue, so dear to the heart of Dr. André Hellegers, may be enhanced.

NOTES

[1] The Catholic University of Louvain (Belgium), The Catholic University of Italy (Milan), Georgetown University (Washington, D.C.), The Pontifical Gregorian University (Rome), The University of Santo Thomas (Manila), and the Borja Institute for Bioethics (Barcelona).

BIBLIOGRAPHY

Abel, F., Boné, E., and Harvey, J. C. (eds.): 1988, *Human Life: Its Beginnings and Development*, L' Harmattan, Paris.

Demmer, K.: 1988, Orientierungsversuche auf schwierigen feld, *Herder Korrespondenz* 42, 438–441.

John XXIII.: 1962, 'Discourse on the opening of the Second Vatican Council', *Acta Apostolica Sedis* 54, 786–796.

John Paul II.: 1980, 'Allocution to the members of the Italian Society of Internal Medicine and the Italian Society of General Surgery', *Acuta Apostolic Sedis* 72, 1125–1129.

KEVIN Wm. WILDES S. J.

FINITUDE, RELIGION, AND MEDICINE: THE SEARCH FOR MEANING IN THE POST-MODERN WORLD

Medicine and religion are driven by the same fundamental human experience: the experience of finitude. The practice of medicine confronts, again and again, the finite nature of human existence in suffering, sickness, death, and the limits of resources. The confrontation with finitude is also an impetus for the religious experience which seeks to understand the meaning of human life in the face of suffering and death. The dilemmas of medical ethics present a unique meeting place for religion and medicine.

In the pastoral practices and theological traditions of the Roman Catholic Church one finds a religious tradition which has repeatedly addressed the finitude of human life encountered in the dilemmas of medicine. This interplay of medicine and faith has taken place on a number of levels. While Catholic physicians, patients, and their confessors have struggled with moral questions provoked by the practice of medicine, popes, theologians, and bishops have sought systematically to understand the resolution of issues, such as the obligation to prolong life, within the context of Christian theology. Indeed the experience of finitude, confronted in the events of death and dying, has simultaneously challenged both the pastoral and intellectual life of the Church.

Today this area of moral and pastoral theology has a tremendous vitality. With the rapid development and availability of medical technology a host of new issues has arisen in medical practice. Through the development of medical technology, for example, we are able to sustain mechanically the lives of patients who just a few years ago would have died. We now must address, in new circumstances, ancient moral questions about our obligations to treat the dying. Such challenges mean that we need to draw from our tradition and rearticulate it in order to address the medical issues of our contemporary world.

The vitality of this area of theology has led to the development of this book. The essays in Part One, written by prominent Catholic physicians, provide the medical background for understanding central moral dilemmas facing contemporary physicians. The essays of Part Two outline the

1

K.Wm. Wildes (ed.), Birth, Suffering and Death, 1–7.
© 1992 *Kluwer Academic Publishers. Printed in the Netherlands.*

foundations of a Catholic understanding and perspective on human life while the essays of Part Three address particular moral issues raised by the events of death and dying.

In the first part the essays explore general medical issues, which provoke discussions of ethical issues. These essays are offered as an informed basis for moral reflection and to illuminate moral discussion by delineating the scope of medical issues confronting contemporary medical practices in the care of patients who are dying. At both ends of the spectrum of human life, the development and availability of technology make it possible to sustain life where it was previously impossible. Robert Cefalo examines medical problems and dilemmas of often tragic dimensions which confront those who care for fetal life while John Harvey sets out the medical issues confronting those who care for the frail elderly. Cefalo illustrates how the development of medical technology allows us the opportunity to diagnose illnesses and congenital malformation before birth leaving the physician, patient, and family with a wide array of choices in treatment which, in turn, often present moral conflicts for those involved. Harvey shows that the health of the elderly is also affected by technology. However, Harvey also points out that the health of the elderly is affected not only by medicine but also by economic and social factors which present new challenges for health care policy.

Ours is an age when moral concerns about the treatment and care for the dying are raised not only in cases of the very young or very old. After a decade of the AIDS epidemic we are confronted with questions about death and the care for the dying in populations where it is usually infrequent: the young and those in the early middle years of their lives. The ethical and policy discussions which surround AIDS and HIV infection are often complicated by medical misinformation. To address this difficulty Edwin Cassem examines the medical issues related to HIV infection. His essay reviews the nature of HIV as a retrovirus, how it presents itself in clinical practice, and the issues it raises for health care workers. Finally, Porter Storey's essay describes the technology involved in feeding and hydrating of patients. Storey's essay serves to familiarize the reader with the technology so that one can better understand the financial, psychological, social, and spiritual costs such treatments can entail.

In the face of suffering men and women, our technological prowess and the limits of health care resources, the moral and public questions occasioned by medicine often concern how we should deploy our technological capabilities. To answer such questions concretely we must articulate our moral and religious understanding of human life. It is within our general understanding of the meaning and purpose of human life that we make our moral and medical choices. It is here also that we recognize the difficulties in moral reflection raised by the development and availability of medical technology are not the only driving force in the contemporary discussion of medical issues in Roman Catholic moral theology. In articulating its understanding of human life the Church encounters an intellectual crisis in the West which affects the Roman Catholic Church and its moral theology (Neuhaus, 1987). As we come to discuss the issues of bioethics today we quickly grasp that there is a wide array of responses to these questions. This experience of moral pluralism, and the inability to speak in terms of a more fundamental, content-full universal narrative is a new challenge for the Church and Western culture.

The culture of the West, since the betrothal of Church and State by Constantine, has been predominantly Christian in its moral outlook. This once powerful cultural vision has, however, been fragmented (MacIntyre, 1981; Engelhardt, 1986) and the West seems to be moving towards de-Christianization (Rahner, 1981). The Church now speaks and acts in a secular, morally pluralistic culture which has many moral voices (Engelhardt, 1991). In the face of such cultural changes it becomes crucial for traditions, such as Catholicism, to reinterpret and rearticulate them-selves so that they can understand themselves and speak to others (MacIntyre, 1988, 1990). The challenge of rearticulating the Roman Catholic moral tradition arises just as health care policy confronts challenges of rising costs and the possibilities unleased by new tech-nologies.

The second part of this book is a collection of essays which set out some of the theological perspectives of the Catholic moral tradition. This section outlines fundamental perspectives for understanding the tradition and responding to contemporary medical developments. Our responses to the medical issues raised in the first section of the book will be shaped by our theological perspectives as Catholics. Among the difficulties one finds are fundamental ambiguities. Frequently the same words are used though their meanings may vary dramatically. Put another way, the melody may sound vaguely familiar but the performance renders it unidentifiable. In addressing the issues raised in this book people will often speak of the "value" or "sanctity" of human life. However, as one listens to the deployment of such language it becomes clear that, while using the same words, people often speak past one another. A challenge to be met is one of clarity in meaning.

The articles by Autiero, Ashley, and Wildes set out the broad framework of the Roman Catholic understanding of the significance of human life. These articles examine the theological context (Autiero, Ashley) for the "sacredness" of human life and the philosophical implications (Wildes) of such a perspective in terms of our obligations to sustain human life. Benedict Ashley explores a model of Christian stewardship in order to understand our responsibility towards our own life and that of others. Antonio Autiero examines the theological basis for the language of the "sanctity" of life while Kevin Wildes sets out a conceptual scheme for understanding biological life and personal life. Diana Bader and Paul Schotsmans draw out the social implications of a Catholic understanding of life and stewardship. Bader develops the implications of a Christian view of sharing responsibility in caring for the dying. She sketches both a theoretical understanding and the practical implications of "mutual support" for one another – particularly those who are dying. Schotsmans explores the implications of a relationship of mutual support for the practice of medicine. The collection of essays included in the second section lays out the conceptual framework which has shaped the Church's moral tradition in medical ethics and respond to contemporary medical ethics.

There is a long tradition in the West, articulated by Aristotle, that ethics is practical wisdom. After all the discussions and investigations about the "moral life", the nature of the "good life", or the interpretation of the "natural law", one is still faced with very practical questions of moral choice. In viewing the moral life as part of practical wisdom, this book would be incomplete without addressing some of the concrete moral questions often confronted in suffering and death. The third part of the book is a collection of essays which seeks to address such particular moral quandaries in contemporary medicine. Kevin O'Rourke, John Paris, and Thomas Bole examine practical issues, such as pain relief, artificial feeding and hydration, and the extent of obligations to care for the dying, which arise in treating patients from the perspective of the Catholic faith. In responding to the issues they deploy the principle of double effect and the distinction of ordinary-extraordinary means. Kevin O'Rourke examines issues of pain relief with lethal effects. In this he re-examines a staple of Roman Catholic moral theology – the principle of double effect. John Paris summarizes and gives an overview of the Catholic tradition's view regarding the feeding and hydration of persistently vegetative patients. Finally, Thomas Bole explores the relationships of resource allocation to the ordinary-extraordinary distinction. In so doing Bole illustrates the vitality of the tradition in addressing contemporary issues in the care of patients and the stewardship of health care resources.

Alasdair MacIntyre has written extensively on the post modern condition and communal traditions (MacIntyre, 1988, 1990). For MacIntyre the ability of a tradition to respond to new problems indicates the vitality of the tradition. Such reinterpretations can take place in at least two ways. On the one hand there is reflection and reinterpretation directed to the daily practices of a tradition and the choices in terms of which the tradition is lived. On the other hand there is reflection on the tradition's relationship to contemporary issues. This book, this series, in addressing issues in bioethics attempts to reflect in both ways. The book, and series, stand as a sign of a tradition that remains vital in confronting the issues of the contemporary world.

Any attempt to reinterpret the tradition of a community, so that it might address the concerns of the contemporary world, will have to bring together, in some fashion, the intellectual and spiritual tradition of the community with the realities and questions of the world. This book includes two appendices which are central documents of the Roman Catholic moral tradition in medical ethics: Pope Pius XII's allocution "The Prolongation of Life" and the Congregation for the Doctrine of the Faith's "Declaration on Euthanasia". The documents are central to the moral tradition of the Church and any attempt to reinterpret that tradition.

To remain vital a tradition must also understand the contemporary world which it inhabits. Even if a community should choose to reject the world and withdraw from it, the community still, nonetheless, has an understanding of the world. An essential element for addressing the moral dilemmas of bioethics is an adequate understanding of the challenges of modern medical practice (McCormick, 1984; McCormick, 1989; Pellegrino and Thomasma, 1981). Central to this volume, indeed the conception of this series, is the goal of bringing together a clear understanding of contemporary medical dilemmas within Catholic moral theology and philosophy. This understanding is a necessary element, not a peripheral nicety, for moral discourse. Indeed the Roman Catholic tradition of moral theology and philosophy has woven together both the rational and the empirical. In the Roman Catholic tradition there is a natural inclination to seek to understand not only moral principles but also the circumstances of moral dilemmas. For example, Lateran IV exhorts confessors to be like skilled physicians and inquire into the circumstances of the penitent (Denzinger and Schonmetzer, #813). Aquinas wrote of the need to understand the circumstances of persons, times, and place in moral evaluation (*Summae Theologica*, I–II, q.18, aa. 10–11). To address the challenges of contemporary bioethics one must understand what they are. We must know both the tradition and the circumstances in which the tradition is lived out. We learn then in two directions. We not only learn about the issues confronting contemporary bioethics and medical practice, but we also learn and develop in our understanding of our tradition of moral theology (Mahoney, 1987).

In this twofold process of learning we better equip ourselves, as Church, for the stresses and demands of a secular world. In a secular world, committed to no particular ideology of the good life for human beings, there will be constant challenges for those who hold a particular vision to be canonical for human life and flourishing. Faced with competing views of the good life, or with people who hold but fragments of values they do not understand, it will be imperative for those who live in a tradition to understand their heritage so that it may be responsive to new challenges and needs, and so be preserved.

The more one comes to understand the richness and nuances of moral traditions and communities, such as Catholicism, the more one comes to recognize the moral impoverishment of secular society. Again the themes of finitude and loss return. The human experience of finitude and loss, often encountered in medicine and religious faith, is encountered in the realm of moral discourse. As the cases of bioethics are discussed within a tradition rich in values, concepts, moral heroes, and moral language, one senses the poverty of the secular context of bioethics.

BIBLIOGRAPHY

Denzinger, H. and Schonmetzer, A.: 1962, *Enchiridion Symbolorum*, Herder, New York

Engelhardt, H. T.: 1991, *Bioethics and Secular Humanism: The Search for a Common Morality*, SCM Press, London.

Engelhardt, H. T.: 1986, *The Foundations of Bioethics*, Oxford University Press, New York.

MacIntyre, A.: 1981, *After Virtue: A Study in Moral Theory*, University of Notre Dame Press, Notre Dame, Indiana.

MacIntyre, A.: 1990, *Three Rival Versions of Moral Enquiry*, University of Notre

Dame Press, Notre Dame, Indiana.
MacIntyre, A.: 1988, *Whose Justice? Which Rationality?*, University of Notre Dame Press, Notre Dame, Indiana.
Mahoney, J.: 1987, *The Making of Moral Theology*, Clarendon Press, Oxford.
McCormick, R.: 1984, *Health and Medicine in the Catholic Tradition*, Crossroad Publishing Company, New York
McCormick, R.: 1989, 'Moral argument in Christian ethics' in McCormick (ed.), *The Critical Calling*, Georgetown University Press, Washington, D. C., pp. 47–70.
Neuhaus, R. J.: 1987, *The Catholic Moment: The paradox of the Church in the Postmodern World*, Harper and Row, San Francisco.
Pellegrino, E. and D. Thomasma: 1981, *A Philosophical Basis of Medical Practice*, Oxford University Press, New York.
Rahner, K.: 1981, 'The future of the Church and the Church of the future' in *Concern for the Church, Theological Investigations*, Vol. XX, Crossroad, N. Y.

MEDICAL BACKGROUND AND ETHICAL ISSUES

ROBERT C. CEFALO

EDGES OF LIFE: THE CONSEQUENCES OF PRENATAL ASSESSMENT, DIAGNOSIS, AND TREATMENT

INTRODUCTION

Of the approximately 3.5 million infants born alive in the United States each year, 4–6% enter neonatal critical care nurseries. The majority is admitted either for major congenital anomalies or low birth weight. Recent advances in maternal-fetal medicine and neonatology have contributed to dramatic decreases in mortality and morbidity. Therefore, a child born with major congenital anomalies or with low birth weight is much more likely to survive today.

When a prenatal diagnosis is made of major congenital anomalies or grand multifetal pregnancies, several factors must be considered: the suffering of the family, the child, and all professionals involved; and the financial burden on the family and on society. These factors have led some to believe that it may be ethically acceptable to routinely perform prenatal screening for congenital anomalies, to terminate a pregnancy, or to perform multifetal pregnancy reduction. Others argue that routine prenatal screening for fetal anomalies and the termination of any pregnancy is unethical and morally wrong.

This paper addresses fetal assessment, prenatal diagnosis and treatment of severe congenital malformations, selective termination of a twin pregnancy with one lethal malformation, and multiple pregnancy reduction (Berkowitz, 1990). Also discussed is the relationship of ethical principles to recent diagnostic advances and medical decision making.

BACKGROUND

Four to six percent of all infants are born with some genetic disorders and fetal malformations. Congenital anomalies are the leading cause of infant mortality. Roughly half of these conditions are minor, but the remainder are major and many are lethal. In approximately 50% of all human birth defects, the cause remains unknown. In about 10% the cause is believed to be environmental, such as maternal infection, drug ingestion, maternal

11

K.Wm. Wildes (ed.), Birth, Suffering and Death, 11–31.
© 1992 *Kluwer Academic Publishers. Printed in the Netherlands.*

fever, or poor placentation leading to an abnormal intrauterine environment.

Ten percent of congenital malformations are inherited according to Mendelian principles of genetics. Most congenital malformations with a genetic basis are polygenic or multifactorial and typically involve a single organ such as the heart (6–8/1000 births), the kidney (4/1000 births), or the neural tube (2/1000 births). Other genetic conditions consist of 0.5% for unbalanced chromosomal abnormalities (e.g., trisomy 21, 13, or 18), and 1% for single gene defects (e.g., Tay Sachs, muscular dystrophy, cystic fibrosis).

The prenatal diagnosis of some structural malformations can be made with high resolution ultrasound starting as early as 10 to 12 weeks gestation. Amniotic fluid or maternal serum alphafetoprotein assessment for the detection of open neural tube defects and other specific anomalies can be made at 16–18 weeks. Cytogenetic analysis of cultured amniotic fluid cells may be obtained at 15–16 weeks. Cytogenetic analysis of cultured amniotic fluid cells may be obtained at 15–16 weeks; chorionic villus sampling for cytogenetic analysis can begin at 9–11 weeks. The results of 6,033 patients who had successful chorionic villus sampling indicated a cytogenetic diagnosis was made in 99.6%, utilizing either the direct method (results in 48 hours) or the culture method (results in 5–7 days) (Rhoads et al., 1989). Fetal cord blood sampling can be performed at 14–16 weeks for both cytogenetic and biochemical analysis utilizing sophisticated biochemical or DNA fragment analysis for the detection of inheritable diseases.

Recently reported was the biopsy of a single cell of an *in vitro* human preimplantation embryo at 6–8 cell stage. The cell biopsy was done for sex determination in fetuses at high risk for X-linked diseases such as Lesch-Nyhan, Duchenne muscular dystrophy, and X-linked mental retardation. Two female embryos from which cells were taken and then biopsied were then transferred to the uterus and were growing normally as determined by ultrasound at 22 weeks (Handyside et al., 1990).

The unfertilized oocyte obtained from standard treatment for infertility has undergone polymerose chain reaction amplification of the DNA sequence of the 1st polar body. This amplification was done to determine if the oocyte carried the defective gene for sickle cell disease or if the defect was absent (Monk, M. and Holding, C., 1990). There is a 50% chance sickle cell disease will be transmitted if an oocyte with a defective gene is fertilized. This amplification technique was reported to be successful and would obviate many of the ethical concerns of biopsy of fertilized cells. In the future, genetic testing of biopsied cells at the 6–8 cell stage may be possible for the definitive diagnosis and possible gene therapy of diseases such as cystic fibrosis, thalassemia and Duchenne muscular dystrophy. Under development is the harvesting of fetal cells and the diagnosis of biochemical defects in the fetus from maternal blood.

Some of the above methods are completely safe and efficacious, while others are investigative and carry risk. So far, ultrasound is without evidence of detectable risks to the mother or fetus. The risk of fetal loss related to amniocentesis has been placed around 0.5%. Chorionic villus sampling is 98% efficacious and appears to introduce an approximately 1% fetal loss risk (Rhoads *et al.*, 1989). Fetal blood sampling has a 1–1.5% fetal loss rate. Preimplantation and oocyte biopsy and diagnosis is still investigative at this time (Handyside *et al.*, 1990; Monk and Holding, 1990).

In the United States today, approximately 50,000 women undergo genetic amniocentesis annually; approximately 5,000 have chorionic villus sampling per year. Most physicians do not place as a condition for amniocentesis or chorionic villus sampling that the patient be willing to terminate the pregnancy. The patient should be free to do what she wishes based upon the information from the test, the evaluation of the information received from the physician, and the patient's own religious and cultural beliefs.

Prenatal screening with amniocentesis is not just performed for the woman age 35 or above who has an increased risk of bearing a child with a serious abnormality. In a recent survey, 76% of geneticists in the United States would perform a prenatal diagnosis for a woman of 25 years of age upon her request with no medical indication. Other geneticists would attempt to dissuade, refer, or refuse the patient under age 35 (Fletcher and Wertz, 1987). One of the main arguments for amniocentesis at any age is the fact that 75–80% of the infants born with trisomy 21 (Down Syndrome) in the United States are born to women less than 35 years old (Fletcher and Wertz, 1987 p. 17–18). Two arguments against genetic amniocentesis at any age are the potential harm to the fetus and the constraint of limited resources (Fletcher and Wertz).

PRENATAL DIAGNOSIS OF SUSPECTED ABNORMALITIES

When a patient is referred with a suspected congenital malformation *in utero*, high resolution and dynamic ultrasound may reassure the patient that everything appears normal. Most studies associated with prenatal diagnosis are normal or negative, thus relieving a significant anxiety. While there is benefit in learning that the fetus appears normal, the physician should not overlook the potential anxiety from false positive tests or reassurance from false negative tests. Although truth and knowledge may bring power, they also mandate decision making. At times, the amount of information given to parents is awesome and adds an extra burden to their lives. If a pregnant patient, who is not at risk, participates in a screening procedure and the fetus turns out to be normal, anxiety and stress are still created. Should there be an abnormality, the parents should receive information as to the possible diagnosis, prognosis, potential treatment modalities, and prospective prenatal and perinatal planning. The physician and the patient must realize that medicine is an inexact science. Many times limitations in assigning a short- or long-term prognosis result from lack of experience in dealing with the specifics of the maternal-fetal dyad because the fetus does not exist in isolation of the mother or the family.

It is imperative that the physician remain up-to-date because of the availability of new and almost daily-changing methods for the anatomical and biochemical evaluation of the fetus. With these modalities, the prenatal recognition of severe abnormalities is over 90%. Fetal therapies are being investigated for some nonlethal malformations. Successful neonatal therapy has been enhanced by the *in utero* diagnosis of nonlethal abnormalities. Ultrasonography can demonstrate structural and functional defects and is a widely accepted technique for visualizing the fetus. In addition to diagnosing congenital malformations of many organ systems with certainty, ultrasound allows for an analysis of the progression of certain anomalies such as hydronephrosis and hydrocephalus. There has also been ultrasound documentation of regression or resolution of certain abnormalities. Specific fetal heart defects are now being diagnosed because of the development of new ultrasound doppler flow techniques previously used for postnatal diagnoses.

Fetal blood sampling and amniocentesis have utilized newer methods to analyze fetal karyotype by examining DNA fragments in fetal cells. Fetal blood sampling allows for rapid karyotyping (7–10 days versus 3 weeks from amniocentesis). When DNA sequencing occurs for the entire human genome for specific gene defects, diagnosis of every known genetic disease will be possible as early as 6–8 weeks' gestation. In addition to amniocentesis, chorionic villus sampling at 9–11 weeks can assist in the diagnosis of chromosomal abnormalities.

Prenatal assessment of the fetus can include those at high and low risk. If a family is known to have a carrier of a disease, the fetus could be identified as high risk. Diseases such as Tay Sachs, phenylketonuria, hemophilia, muscular dystrophies, cystic fibrosis, and common hemoglobinopathies can be diagnosed from a sampling of fetal blood. Prenatal assessment of the fetus at low risk can be performed by a screening test. Maternal serum alphafetoprotein (MSAFP) is elevated in a fetus with an open neural tube defect. A low MSAFP is associated with an increased risk for a chromosomal anomaly such as trisomy 21; currently the combination of a low MSAFP, a low maternal estriol, and a high level of human chorionic gonadotropin can detect about 60% of affected pregnancies, whereas genetic amniocentesis for the women over 35 years will detect only 15% of all Down Syndrome fetuses prenatally. A finding of abnormalities in the level of alphafetoprotein in the amniotic fluid also assists in the diagnosis of neural tube defects or ventral wall defects such as omphalocele and gastroschisis.

Prenatal diagnosis is therapeutic in selective cases; further damage can be prevented by intervention such as drainage of an obstructed organ (e.g., the bladder in cases of urethral obstruction) (Globus, 1985). At present there is no *in utero* treatment to correct bowel atresias, omphalocele, meningomyelocele, and unilateral dysplastic kidney. The treatment of Rh isoimmunization of the fetus by intraabdominal or intraumbilical cord transfusion is a well-accepted standard of care. In the future there may be surgery on a partially removed and replaced fetus for the repair of a known defect such as diaphragmatic hernia or cardiac anomaly. There are some treatments that are still investigative that may involve medical intervention *in utero*. Such interventions may include treatment of specific fetal arrhythmias by the administration of antiarrhythmic cardiac drugs to the mother and treatment of known fetal vitamin-dependent enzyme deficiencies.

Prenatal diagnosis allows preparation for the birth at a perinatal center equipped and prepared for the immediate neonatal care of the sick infant. There are many examples of infants whose survival was directly aided by antenatal diagnosis of a malformation such as gastroschisis or diaphragmatic hernia. It is clear that the physician has the opportunity to diagnose and occasionally treat the fetus as a patient, and that the task of the physician is to ensure the health of both mother and child.

The prenatal risk assessment of the fetus and diagnosis of a birth defect early in pregnancy is not a search and destroy mission. For those fetuses deemed low risk by reason of maternal family history and current pregnancy findings, prenatal diagnosis need not be considered. For the fetus at risk or for the mother who wishes more information about her pregnancy, a screening test such as MSAFP or a diagnostic ultrasound, may be considered. In the United States, approximately 60% of pregnancies have at least one ultrasound. Most of these relate to uncertainty about dates. No matter what method, prenatal diagnosis allows for full and open discussion of the data, evaluation of the options, and time for the prospective parents to understand the implications of the diagnosis and the possibilities and limitations of medical technology (Clark and DeVore, 1989). However, there are a number of situations that involve the unfortunate dilemma of either termination of pregnancy or parental preparation for a handicapped child. Assisting the parents requires not only an evaluation of the abnormality but also respect for moral and ethical decisions for all involved in the decision making process. The decision making process may be different for a couple with a previous malformed child than for a couple who receives potentially "bad" information from a routine screening program. In addition, the couple at risk for a serious fetal anomaly or disease, by reason of parental carrier state family history or the previous birth of an affected child, may consider prenatal diagnosis their only avenue for considering pregnancy and thus consider prenatal assessment and diagnosis as "prolife" either by reason of prenatal preparation for the birth of another handicapped child or the opportunity for exercising options.

SPECIFIC EXAMPLES OF ETHICAL CHALLENGES IN PERINATAL
MEDICINE ASSOCIATED WITH CONGENITAL MALFORMATIONS

A. *Fetal Hydrocephalus*

The prenatal diagnosis of fetal hydrocephalus is usually made by ultrasound performed because the maternal uterine size is greater than the gestational dates. For many years, the standard of care in patients with a hydrocephalic fetus has been neonatal cerebrospinal fluid shunt surgery. The post surgical survival rate changed from 44% reported in 1973 to 86% reported in 1982 (Mealy *et al.*, 1973; McCullough and Balzar-Martin, 1982). If surgery is not performed, the survival rate is less than 10%. Although the reports did not exclude other handicapping conditions, of the survivors who received surgical treatment, 28–40% were severely handicapped and 19–25% were mildly handicapped with evidence of mental retardation, vision abnormalities and seizures (McCullough and Balzar-Martin, 1982; Mealy *et al.*, 1973). However, the long-term prognosis of infants with isolated hydrocephalus varies and there is potential for normal development and intelligence (Chervenak *et al.*, 1985; Lorber, J., 1981; Strong, 1987). If the diagnosis of hydrocephalus is made before 30 weeks gestation and there is evidence of rapid progression, an *in utero* verticuloamniotic shunt has been considered. The results of these shunts have not been overwhelmingly positive (Chervenak *et al.*, 1985). There is a world-wide moratorium on the use of *in utero* shunt therapy. With evidence of rapidly progressive fetal hydrocephalus it is advisable to wait until 30 weeks' gestation before delivering the fetus. The survival rate of fetuses born at 30 weeks is almost 90% and, if necessary, neonatal surgery can be performed with a high degree of safety and success (Cochrane, 1982).

Upon the decision to effect delivery, usually because of severe progressive hydrocephalus, maternal and fetal concerns are considered. The first approach is the recommendation of a cesarean delivery in order to avoid fetal trauma. Most patients will accept this recommendation. If the mother refuses a cesarean delivery, an alternate choice would be a vaginal delivery after induction of labor. At 30 weeks gestation and with fetal hydrocephalus, there is a high degree of failure of induction of labor, which requires a subsequent cesarean delivery. If the mother also refuses the induction of labor option, the hydrocephalus more than likely would progress and a cephalocentesis could be performed with the hope of a vaginal delivery (Chervenak *et al.*, 1985; Chervenak and McCullough, 1987). Cephalocentesis is performed with a needle placed through the maternal abdomen into the fetal brain with drainage of the excess fluid and decompression of the fetal head (Chervenak *et al.*, 1985). There is minimal potential for maternal trauma either from the procedure or the subsequent vaginal delivery. However, many times cephalocentesis and subsequent vaginal delivery involve a stillbirth or neonatal death secondary to the fetal trauma. The use of cephalocentesis is usually reserved for *severe* hydrocephalus in which there is maternal refusal of a cesarean, induction of labor, or where there is the possibility of uterine rupture resulting from overdistention of the uterus. Cephalocentesis is also performed on a fetus with severe malformations in addition to hydrocephalus.

In the presence of severe hydrocephalus without any other debilitating anomalies, a cesarean delivery and a *neonatal* ventriculoperitoneal or atrial shunting is efficacious. The mother may refuse the cesarean for many complex reasons, such as fear of a major surgical operation or concerns about caring for a handicapped child with a potential for mental retardation. If the mother refuses the cesarean, the physician and the patient are confronted with a difficult decision that involves both ethical and medical duties and obligations (Chervenak and McCullough, 1985 and 1987).

An essential principle of medicine is providing the best possible care for both the pregnant woman and the child while balancing the benefits and risks to each. The beneficence principle of medicine dictates the use of clinical intervention to provide the greatest benefit with the least risk (Beauchamp and McCullough, 1984; Chervenak and McCullough, 1975). This principle could apply to both the mother and physician to avoid harm to the fetus. In addition, the woman who decides to maintain her pregnancy is morally charged and entrusted with promoting the "best interests" of the viable or potentially viable fetus and therefore has beneficence-based obligations (Chervenak and McCullough, 1984; Chervenak and McCullough, 1975). On the other hand, the beneficence principle also guides the physician to avoid potential harm and suffering by the mother. In addition, there is the autonomy principle, which may be the basis for maternal decisions and which obligates a physician to treat the mother based on what she perceives is in her own best interest (Beauchamp and McCullough, 1984). However, the physician is not totally free of fetal obligations because of maternal autonomy. Both respect for autonomy and beneficence-based principles generate duties and moral obligations that portend for a potential conflict between physician and the patient (Chervenak and McCullough, 1985).

More than 60% of infants with hydrocephalus have other neural tube anomalies and cardiac anomalies not so readily apparent by prenatal diagnosis (Chervenak *et al.*, 1985; Strong, 1987). Even with isolated hydrocephalus the incidence of mental retardation is greater than expected (Chervenak *et al.*, 1985; Lorber, 1981; McCullough and Balzar-Martin,

1982). Although it is possible for the child with treated hydrocephalus to develop normally, it is impossible to predict with certainty which fetuses with hydrocephalus will have developmental delays or other anomalies (Chervenak *et al.*, 1985). The fact that the mother has refused termination of the pregnancy prior to her knowledge of fetal hydrocephalus implies her feeling of maternal "duty" to her fetus; by continuing with the pregnancy she is expressing free choice (Engelhardt, 1985).

The physician should present a balanced evaluation to the mother both from a scientific point of view and regarding the moral obligations generated by a particular situation (Strong, 1987). In the case of a viable fetus with hydrocephalus and no other obvious anomaly, the physician should attempt to convince the woman that her ethical obligation is consistent with the professional recommendation to perform a cesarean delivery for the sole benefit of the child. The American College of Obstetricians and Gynecologists (ACOG), in a statement in 1987, recognized there may be a conflict when the pregnant woman's opinion and decision do not concur with the recommendations of the physician (ACOG, 1987). The ACOG statement suggests that the physician should try to understand the values and beliefs that lead the patient to her decision. In hopes of a better understanding between the physician and the patient, both should seek consultation from a variety of sources including geneticists, pediatric surgeons, neonatologists, spiritual advisors, and social workers. Ultimately, the pregnant woman may decide that having a cesarean delivery is a greater risk than the potential benefit to the fetus. If there is persistent conflict between the medical recommendation and the patient's wishes, consultation with the institutional ethics committee may provide a vehicle for resolution. Actions of coercion to obtain a court order to perform a procedure on the mother for the sole benefit of the fetus could violate a woman's autonomy and fracture the trust relationship between the patient and the physician. Therefore, the physician should present an approach that considers the welfare of the fetus, the maternal health needs, and the woman's declared values and freedom of choice. Usually the woman will make a decision on behalf of the fetus. If the woman fails to consent to a cesarean delivery, the physician should not abandon the patient; in such a case, the physician should refer the patient or should try cephalocentesis to attempt a vaginal delivery unless this cannot be performed in good conscience. Strong advocates seeking court authorization prior to performing a decompression procedure to avoid any possibility of misunderstanding of the law potential criminal accusation (Strong, 1987).

Hydrocephalus is often associated with other abnormalities such as bilateral renal agenesis, pulmonary hypoplasia with a thanatophoric dwarf, trisomy 13 or 18, or alobar holoprosencephaly (absent cerebral hemispheres). These abnormalities have fairly certain prognoses, severe physical and mental handicaps and early death. The gravity of such outcomes may free both physician and pregnant woman from Engelhardt's fiduciary argument and the beneficence principle (Chervenak and McCullough, 1987; Engelhardt, 1985; Strong, 1987). In the presence of such severe anomalies, cephalocentesis may be performed to allow for decreased maternal trauma from the cesarean or a vaginal delivery. An *indirect* effect may be the demise of t:he fetus but the direct intent is to decrease the harm to the mother. In such cases, the physician's moral obligation is greater to the pregnant women. In the case of hydrocephalus with life-threatening anomalies, the physician may justifiably make certain recommendations: (1) vaginal, rather than cesarean delivery; (2) cephalocentesis, if necessary to enable vaginal delivery; (3) no intervention upon signs of fetal distress; and (4) intrapartum electronic monitoring of the fetal heart rate.

In every case where fetal hydrocephalus is diagnosed, a thorough evaluation of the fetus should be performed, including fetal karyotype, to look for other anomalies. Consultation with neonatologists and neurosurgeons is necessary to ensure that the most current opinion be given to the parents. The degree of hydrocephalus, gestational age of the fetus, and potential therapeutic options must be presented to the parents in a nondirective manner.

B. Anencephaly

In 1982, a tidal wave of concern was precipitated by the birth of an infant with Down Syndrome and esophageal atresia, and the parent's subsequent decision to withhold treatment. The Baby Doe Law, as passed in 1985, in the Federal Register defines medical neglect as the failure to respond to an infant's life-threatening condition by providing treatment (including appropriate nutrition, hydration, and medication) which, in the treating physician or physicians' reasonable medical judgment, will most likely be effective in ameliorating or correcting all such conditions. Three separately sufficient exceptions to the rules are: (1) the infant is chronically and irreversibly comatose; (2) the provisions of such treatment would merely prolong dying, not be effective in correcting all the infant's life-threatening conditions or otherwise be futile in terms of the survival of the infant; or (3) the provision of such treatment would be virtually futile in terms of the survival of the infant, and the treatment itself under such circumstances would be inhumane (U.S. Department of Health and Human Services, 1985).

One example of an exception would be a child born with *anencephaly*, where only comfort treatment should be given. This defect is regarded as resulting from nonclosure of the neural tube. The human neural folds that form in the brain normally complete their closure by the 24th day postconception in the human. Anencephaly is considered to arise prior to this time. Anencephaly includes lack of development of both cerebral hemispheres and hypothalamus, incompletely developed pituitary and skull, altered facial features rendering a grotesque appearance, and abnormalities of the cervical vertebrae.

Until recently in the United States, approximately 2,000–3,000 anencephalics were born each year. This number has dropped dramatically because of maternal serum alphafetoprotein screening programs and subsequent termination of pregnancy. When termination of pregnancy is not elected, only approximately 50% of anencephalics are born alive. Of these, approximately two-thirds will die in the first 24 hours, with the additional one-third expiring within one week. Most live born anencephalics die from respiratory failure after repeated episodes of bradycardia and asphyxia. Anencephaly is a uniformly fatal disease. The frequency of anencephaly differs among western countries and is stated to be from 0.5 to 1.0% of all pregnancies. In the United States, the frequency of the anencephaly is six times higher in whites than in blacks. This malformation is frequently observed in Caucasian populations of the British Isles, India, and Egypt, and especially in Iran (4%). An emphasis is placed on the frequency of anencephaly in Catholics of Irish descent. The female sex predominates; the anencephalic population as only 20 to 30% of anencephalics are males. The maternal serum alphafetoprotein levels are in high concentrations in anencephaly, both in the mother's blood and in the amniotic fluid. Prenatal diagnosis can be made with certainty by ultrasound examination.

The question of termination of pregnancy in a diagnosed malformation that is definitely combined with a limited life span has been debated over many years. The anencephalic fetus can die either during labor and delivery or, if born alive, should not be given treatment that would prolong dying. In this way, the newborn is allowed to die a natural death.

With anencephaly a potential for cognitive function never exists. Therefore, it may be morally permissible to terminate the pregnancy if the fetus is afflicted with a condition that is incompatible with postnatal survival for more than a few weeks, and if it is characterized by the total or virtual absence of cognitive functions. If the anencephalic never develops the neurological substrate necessary for even minimal human sentience, then the anencephalic lacks the necessary condition for human personhood (Cefalo and Engelhardt, 1989).

Those who advise or chose to terminate pregnancy in which anencephaly has been clearly established cannot be said to be acting in a way that is morally wrong. Furthermore, the use of anencephalics after delivery, as a source of organs and tissues for transplantation is not a violation of personal dignity (Cefalo and Engelhardt, 1989).

C. Selective Termination and Multifetal Pregnancy Reduction

If prenatal diagnosis reveals twins, with one affected by a *congenital malformation* that directly affects the health and welfare of the "normal" twin, there are several, options, treatment options, depending on gestational age: (1) continuation of the pregnancy with predictable death of normal twin, (2) preparation for the birth of an abnormal child, (3) termination of the pregnancy despite the presence of a normal twin, or (4) selective feticide of the abnormal fetus. All options have risks, some more than others. Fortunately, the combination of a normal twin and one with a lethal abnormality is rare. Experience is limited in selective termination of one twin with a lethal abnormality.

Usually this diagnosis is made in the second trimester which adds to the risk and emotional difficulty. *In utero* treatment of the anomalous twin may place the healthy twin at risk for unanticipated damage or premature delivery. Prior to fetal viability, the woman has the legal option to abort *both* fetuses.

The various methods reported to terminate the anomalous fetus selectively are investigated with isolated case reports (Rhoads *et al.*, 1989; Alberg *et al.*, 1978; Kerenyi, 1981; Petres and Redwine, 1981; Platt *et al.*, 1983). When a diagnosis is made prior to viability, a hysterotomy and removal of the malformed fetus has been performed, as well as *in utero* interruption of the umbilical cord circulation of the anomalous fetus (Platt *et al.*, 1983). Most of these methods deal with a rare anomaly

(1/35,000 births) known as an acardiac monster in which one of the fetuses is present with multiple major anomalies and without a functional heart. The acardiac twin is perfused by the "donor" heart of the normal twin through placental anastomosis. If the condition were to continue, the mortality rate in the unaffected (donor) twin would be over 50%.

The parents facing the prenatal diagnosis of one twin with a lethal abnormality and one twin with normal development face a complex and tragic dilemma: the choice between risking both twins or ensuring the survival of the healthy one. Because selective termination is rather new, the true risks and benefits are not yet known. The direct lethal injection of a cardiotoxic agent into the anomalous fetus has been reported as a means of termination (Kerenyi and Chitkaro, 1981). There are maternal and fetal risks of infection, including premature delivery. Retention of the dead fetus may be associated with a life-threatening maternal disseminated intravascular coagulation.

Feticide of the anomalous twin may injure or kill the normal fetus and, therefore, more harm than good could occur. If the physician takes no action, there is the risk of doing more harm than good because of the natural consequences of the condition. With the removal of the anomalous twin there is the possibility of enabling the surviving fetus to develop normally. In this case, more good than harm would have been done. Selective termination seems to result in more good and least harm under conditions where one fetus has a known lethal abnormality that is directly affecting the growth and development of the normal twin or jeopardizing the pregnancy by reason of premature labor, polyhydramnios, or other conditions.

In 1986, Redwine and Hays reviewed the world literature of selective birth and added their most recent experience (Redwine and Hays, 1986). The indication for the selective birth in the presence of genetic discordant twins included metabolic disease such as Hurler and Tay Sachs disease, chromosomal abnormalities such as trisomy 21, and inherited diseases such as hemophilia A and thalassemia major. Even though the outcome for the eight surviving twins in the 11 cases was good, the authors caution that surgical procedures such as direct toxic cardiac puncture and air insufflation are new and relatively untested. The 30% fetal loss rate was a result of spontaneous abortion, preterm labor and delivery, and in-trauterine fetal death occurring at varying times after the procedure (Redwine and Hays, 1986).

This experience makes it difficult to counsel parents; regardless, the procedure should only be performed prior to viability and should not be performed for trivial reasons such as sex selection or the desire to "electively" reduce a normal twin or triplet gestation to a singleton pregnancy. Great consideration and reflection should be given to the use of this procedure in the presence of a chromosomal abnormality such as trisomy 21, where the opportunity for sentience and interrelatedness is present. The potential 30% perinatal mortality rate for the surviving normal twin after the procedure and the potential risks to the mother are too great to perform the procedure in a pregnancy that does not have a lethal abnormality in one twin or the presence of pathophysiology in the abnormal twin that directly affects the potential for normal growth and development of the remaining fetus.

Elias and Annas have argued in favor of selective termination of a twin with a genetic abnormality such as Tay-Sachs disease (Elias and Annas, 1987). They outline strict criteria for ethical acceptance in addition to grounding their choice of selective termination on the legality of abortion. The parents must be informed of the lack of experience, potential for complications, and potential loss of the pregnancy as a result of the invasive procedure.

Another bioethical dilemma deals with grand multifetal pregnancies (4,5,6 or more) as a result of ovulation induction treatment of infertility, *in vitro* fertilization, or gamete intrafallopian tube transfer. The spontaneous incidence of twin pregnancy is about 1% and the spontaneous incidence of pregnancies with 3 or more fetuses is very rare. However, with the use of fertility drugs the incidence of twin pregnancies is about 10% of patients and is reported to be 23 % (249/1092) of deliveries from *in vitro* fertilization or gamete intrafallopian tube transfer (Working Party, 1990). Medically induced grand multifetal gestations (4 or more fetuses) occur in 1% of patients despite biochemical and ultrasound monitoring of the patient (Evans *et al.*, 1988). In cases of quadruplets, pentuplets, or sextuplets, the fetal outcomes have been very poor. The study of 1267 assisted conceptions revealed a 24% preterm delivery rate compared to a 6% control rate and a perinatal mortality rate of twice the average rate; both factors were attributable to the high frequency of multiple gestation (Working Party, 1990).

There are recent reports on reduction of multifetal pregnancies to singleton or twin gestation (Dumez and Oury, 1986; Berkowitz *et al.*, 1988; Wapner *et al.*, 1990). If the patient is carrying 4 or more fetuses, there is very little chance that viability will be assured for any one of the fetuses, but it has occurred (Hobbins, 1988). It appears that the perinatal mortality rate for pregnancies with greater than three fetuses is twenty times normal, with a very high prematurity, stillbirth, intrauterine growth retardation, and congenital malformation rate (MacLennon, 1984, pp. 527–538). In addition, there are severe maternal burdens on the circulatory, renal, and endocrine systems. The mother is more likely to have preeclampsia, placenta previa, placental abruption, premature labor, and a very prolonged bed-rest period.

The women with grand multifetal pregnancies could attempt to carry, with prolonged bed-rest, and take the risk of the abnormalities noted above. Alternatively, she could terminate the pregnancy or attempt selective reduction of the grand multifetal gestation to twins or a singleton pregnancy. The methods for selective reduction include a transvaginal and/or transabdominal aspiration of selected fetal amniotic sacs or direct injection of a cardiotoxic agent into the fetal heart or thoracic cavity. Either procedure is difficult, may require several attempts, and is usually performed at 6–12 weeks' gestation. In most reports, the grand multiple pregnancies were reduced to a twin gestation (Berkowitz et al., 1988; Evans et al., 1988; Wapner et al., 1990).

All counseling on the potential outcome of pregnancies with four or more fetuses is tentative at best because virtually nothing but case reports are available. The most extensive experience was that of Wapner et al., who reported in 1990 on the experience of selective reduction in 46 multifetal pregnancies. There were varying indications for the procedure: 34 women with multifetal pregnancies ranging from 6 to 2 prereduction to singleton, twin, or triplet pregnancies; 8 women with congenitally abnormal coexisting fetuses such as thanatophoric twin, neural tube defect, and hydrocephalus and chromosomal abnormalities of 21, 18, 9, 45X position; and 4 women who had triplet or twin pregnancies and would have aborted the pregnancies if selective reduction to a singleton was not performed. There was a 94% survival rate (75/80 fetuses) after selective reduction. Spontaneous abortion and neonatal death accounted for the 6% loss rate. There was a 9.9% intrauterine growth retardation role in the surviving fetuses (Wapner et al., 1990).

It must be stressed that selective reduction of fetuses is still experimental and investigative and can result in abortion, infection, bleeding, premature rupture of membranes and premature delivery, and potential damage to remaining fetuses. Because of limited experience, the safety of the procedure for the remaining fetuses is unknown. There is no question that grand multifetal pregnancy is a serious risk to the mother and the fetuses (MacLennon, 1987). Wapner *et al.*, have instituted a registry of cases to evaluate the outcomes from the procedure. As of early 1990, there have been 246 cases of multifetal pregnancy reduction reported with the subsequent live-delivered fetus (Evans *et al.*, 1989; Evans *et al.*, 1988; Wapner *et al.*, 1990). These surviving infants have not had long-term development studies, but short-term studies indicate that many would have faced certain death by abortion or premature delivery. Close observation of the data and experience is indicated.

Greater medical emphasis must be placed on preventing iatrogenic grand multifetal pregnancies with the use of superovulatory drugs. It is incumbent upon the reproductive societies and their treatments, both the pharmacological and *in vitro* methods, for the protection of the mother and her fetuses from a life threatening situation. The issue of the optimum number of eggs to be fertilized, the optimum number of embryos to be placed in the uterus during one cycle and the potential of freezing storage and subsequent thawing of spare embryos should be discussed openly with the couple prior to the treatment. Multifetal pregnancy reduction and selective termination is a highly emotional and distressing procedure to both the parents and the physician. Much more investigation is needed as to the causes and the natural course of grand multifetal pregnancies particularly in relationship to the rapid advances in perinatology that have recently demonstrated marked reductions in the neonatal mortality of the 600–800 gram infant.

At this time the potential harm and complications of selective termination may be outweighed by the good received when a fetus with a lethal malformation directly or indirectly risks the growth and development of an apparently normal co-existing fetus(es). The legal option of elective termination of pregnancy before viability does not reduce to simple electism the grievous moral option of selective reduction. The reduction or feticide of apparently normal fetuses from a twin or triplet pregnancy to a singleton or the selective reduction of fetuses with nonlethal abnormalities or for a desired sex is not morally or medically justified.

SUMMARY

Currently, we have an unprecedented control over conception, ultrasonic diagnosis, amniocentesis, and fetal blood sampling, all of which allow for more information regarding options about when to plan, manage, or terminate a complicated pregnancy. New technologies and new skills can bring more troubling moral, ethical, and legal conundrums to which there may be no easy answers.

The use of prenatal diagnosis relates to the degree of accuracy, the knowledge of the natural course of the disease, and the potential for therapy. Not all of the technologies are perfect and some will fail, leaving the parents with continued sorrow, pain and emotional stress. We, as a society, must be concerned and move in a deliberate, sensitive manner with much reflection prior to accepting a diagnosis, its natural course, or its therapy as routine. The trends that become the standards must also incorporate tolerance for the physician to act in a way that protects his/her freedom of conscience. The expectations of the patient for the "perfect child" and the pressures from society at times create a climate of societal pressure on the physicians. The physician and the patient are not obligated to act in a way that is against the clear judgment of their conscience. In a similar way, the physician is not obligated to perform a procedure chosen by the patient if the physician believes it is not indicated or is dangerous. If it is "necessary care" and the physician cannot perform the procedure, then the physician is obligated to refer the patient to another experienced physician who may agree with the patient's request (Holder, 1988). With prenatal diagnosis the physician can play many roles with regard to the various degrees of counseling and medical or surgical treatment. At all times there must be respect for the freedom of both the physician and the patient to act according to their own ethical guidelines and cultural beliefs.

Whenever a patient is carrying a fetus with a congenital malformation, the physician should appreciate and recognize the emotional impact, anxiety, guilt, shock, anger, loss of self-esteem, helplessness and vulnerability of both the mother and father. Any of these can lead to depression and disruption of a marriage and family life. Prenatal diagnosis of a severely malformed child necessitates empathy, psycho-social support, both at the time of diagnosis and during the follow-up period, and, most importantly, humanication – i.e., constant communication between all humans involved, which includes the art of listing as well as talking. Prenatal diagnosis of a congenitally malformed fetus is only the beginning of a period of communication that must deal with both the physical and emotional concerns of the patient. Such concerns may be amplified by the ability of the patient-family to understand the information received. Generally, prenatal decisions will require numerous discussions and value judgments. Value judgments will be based on knowledge, experience, and cultural and religious influences. The physician's obligations are both to the mother and her fetus and are developed from the bases of moral beliefs and scientific truth. Prenatal diagnosis and treatment should be offered by methods that are scientifically sound, safe, and effective. Only through balanced argumentation, not extreme views encumbered with emotionalism, can a supportive alliance with the parents be developed. This alliance must include the values cherished by the individual families, both religious and cultural.

There should also be a heightened awareness by the medical profession and the public at large of the importance of preconceptional health in relationship to the potential prevention of congenital malformations. Pregnancy is at least a 12-month event; a prepregnancy health inventory can detect abnormalities that may optimize a positive pregnancy outcome. The patients should be informed in the prepregnancy counseling session of the 4–6% incidence of congenital malformation in liveborn infants. This understanding in the prepregnancy period will help alleviate some of the anxiety and guilt associated with prenatal diagnosis of a fetus with a malformation. It is the duty and obligation of the physician to educate the public and the media of the importance of prepregnancy counseling. Such education would be a major step forward for the understanding of the patient and the understanding by the public of the physician's goal to preserve and dignify life, not to destroy it. Further scientific advances in the diagnosis of defective eggs in the unfertilized state could circumvent much of the ethical problems associated with prenatal diagnosis.

CONCLUSION

An obstetric standard of care should include assessment of the risk status of both the mother and the fetus. If either is at risk, prenatal diagnostic methods may be indicated. After the patient has been fully informed as to the reason and potential outcomes of the screening or diagnostic procedure, she is fully justified in refusing the procedure. If parents exercise this judgment they should not be regarded as irresponsible. Difficult decisions concerning the utilization of prenatal diagnosis procedures should be a team effort and should not rest solely on the patient. The physician should guide the patient through the maps of moral values and principles as they relate to the screening and/or diagnostic procedures. Guiding the patient through the terrain of moral values based on scientific data will lead to clear and rational thinking. Consultation may be necessary so that the short- knowledgeable patient is more likely to make wise choices. The physician should respect the patient's values and cultural beliefs at all times. The patient and the physician should not act in a vacuum.

Unfortunately, prenatal diagnosis is an "afterthought." At times, not enough deliberation and conscious reflection precedes reproduction. However, most pregnancies are normal. The physician's role is not to heighten anxiety but to allay fears; otherwise a worry-well society is created. The parents should understand that despite technological advances, medicine is still an imperfect art and the physician cannot guarantee, or the patient demand, a "perfect" outcome.

BIBLIOGRAPHY

Adams, M. M., Finley, S., Hansen, H. *et al.*: 1981, 'Utilization of prenatal genetic diagnosis in women > 35, United States 1977–1978', *American Journal of Obstetrics and Gynecology* 139, 673–677.

Alberg, A., Metelman, F. and Crantz, M.: 1978, 'Cardiac puncture of a fetus with Hurler's Disease avoiding abortion of the unaffected co-twin', *The Lancet* II, 990.

American College of Obstetricians and Gynecologists Committee Opinion: 1987, 'Patient choice: Maternal and fetal conflict,' (55).

American Medical Association: 1986, 'Current opinion of the Council on the Ethical and Judicial Affairs of the AMA' *Journal of American Medical Association* 2, 16–19.

Beauchamp, T. L. and McCullough, L. B.: 1984, *Medical Ethics: The Moral Responsibilities of Physicians*, Prentice Hall, Englewood Cliffs, New Jersey, 22–51.

Berkowitz, R. L., Lynch, L., Chitkara, V. *et al.*: 1988, 'Selective reduction of multifetal pregnancies in the first trimester', *The New England Journal of Medicine* 318(16), 1043–1045.

Berkowitz, R. L. and Lynch, L.: 1990, 'Selective reduction: An unfortunate misnomer', *Obstetrics and Gynecology* 75, 873–874.

Cefalo, R. C. and Engelhardt, H. T. Jr.: 1989, 'The use of fetal and anencephalic tissue for transplantation', *The Journal of Medicine and Philosophy* 14, 25–29.

Chervenak, F. A., Berkowitz, R. L., Tortora, M. *et al.*: 1985, 'The management of fetal hydrocephalus', *American Journal of Obstetrics and Gynecology* 151, 941–953.

Chervenak, F. A. and McCullough, L. B.: 1985, 'Perinatal ethics: A practical method of analysis of obligations to the mother and fetus', *Obstetrics and Gynecology* 66, 442–446.

Chervenak, F. A. and McCullough, L. B.: 1987, 'Ethical challenges in perinatal medicine: The intrapartum management of pregnancy complicated by fetal hydrocephalus with macrocephaly', *Seminars in Perinatology* 11(3), 232–239.

Clark, S. L. and DeVore, G. R.: 1989, 'Prenatal diagnosis for couples who would not consider abortion', *Obstetrics and Gynecology* 73(6), 1035–1038.

Cochrane, D. D. and Myles, S. T.: 1982, 'Management of intrauterine hydrocephalus', *Journal of Neurosurgery* 57, 590–595.

Dumez, Y. and Oury, J. F.: 1986, 'Method of first trimester selection abortion in multiple pregnancy', *Contributions to Gynecology and Obstetrics* 15, 50–53.

Elias, S. and Annas, G. J.: 1987, *Reproductive Genetics and the Law*, Chicago, Year Book, pp. 123–129.

Engelhardt, H. T. Jr.: 1985, 'Current controversies in obstetrics: Wrongful life and forced fetal surgical procedures', *American Journal of Obstetrics and Gynecology* 151, 313–316.

Evans, M. I., Fletcher, J. C. and Rodeck, C.: 1989, 'Ethical problems in multiple gestation: Selective termination', Section 4, in Evans, Fletcher, Dexler, and Schulman (eds.), *Fetal Diagnosis and Therapy, Science, Ethics and the Law*, J. B. Lippincott Company, Philadelphia, p. 270.

Evans, M. I., Fletcher, J. C., Zador, I. E. *et al.*: 1988, 'Selective first trimester termination in octuplet, and quadruplet pregnancies: Clinical ethical issues', *Obstetrics and Gynecology* 71, 289–296.

Fletcher, J. C. and Wertz, D. C.: 1987, 'Ethical aspects of prenatal diagnosis: Views of U.S. medical geneticists', *Clinics in Perinatology* 14(2), 293–311.

Fuchs, J.: 1983, 'The absoluteness of behavioral moral norms', *Personal Responsibility and Christian Morality*, Georgetown University Press, Washington, D. C., 115–152.

Globus, M. L. (ed.): 1985, 'Fetal therapy', *Seminars in Perinatology* VIX(2), 51–136.

Handyside, A. H., Kontogianni, E. H. and Hardy, K., Winston R. M. L.: 1990, 'Pregnancies from biopsied human preimplantation embryos sexed by Y-specific DNA amplification', *Nature* 344, 768–770.

Henifin, M. S.: 1988, 'Selective termination of pregnancy: A commentary', *Hastings Center Report*, pp. 22–23.

Hobbins, J. C.: 1988, 'Selective reduction: A perinatal necessity?', *The New England Journal of Medicine* 318, 1062–1063.

Holder, A. R.: 1988, 'Selective termination of pregnancy: A commentary', *Hastings Center Report*, pp. 21–22.

Kerenyi, T. D. and Chitkaro, V.: 1981, 'Selective birth in twin pregnancy with discordancy for Down's Syndrome', *The New England of Medicine* 304, 1525.

Kovner, E. M., Cox, W. S. and Vople, J. J.: 1984, 'Development and marked reconstitution of the cerebral mantle after postnatal treatment of hydrocephalus', *Neurology* 34, 840–845.

Ledbetter, D. H., Martin, A. O., Verlinsky, Y. *et al.*: 1990, 'Cytogenetic results of chorionic villus sampling: High success rate and diagnostic accuracy', *American Journal of Obstetrics and Gynecology* 162(2), 495–501.

Lorber, J.: 1981 (suppl), 'The results of early treatment of extreme hydrocephalus', *Med Child Neurol*, 16, 21.

MacLennon, A. H.: 1984, 'Multiple gestations', In Creasy, R. K., Resnick, R. (eds), *Maternal-Fetal Medicine: Principles and Practice*, W. B. Saunders, Philadelphia, pp. 527–538.

McCullough, D. C. and Balzar-Martin, L. A.: 1982, 'Current prognosis overt neonatal hydrocephalus', *Journal of Neurosurgery* 57, 378–383.

Mealy, J. Jr., Gelmar, R. L. and Bubb, M. P.: 1973, 'The prognosis of hydrocephalus overt at birth', *Journal of Neurosurgery* 39, 348–355.

Monk, M. and Holding, C.: 1990, 'Amplification of a B-hemoglobin sequence in individual human oocytes and polar bodies', *The Lancet* 355, 985–988.

Petres, R. E. and Redwine, F. U.: 1981 (letter), 'Selective birth in twin pregnancy', *The New England Journal of Medicine* 305:1218–1219.

Platt, L. D., DeVore, G. R., Bilniarz, A. *et al.*: 1983, 'Antenatal diagnosis of acephalia acardia. A proposed management scheme', *American Journal of Obstetrics and Gynecology* 146, 857–859.

Redwine, F. O. and Hays, P. M.: 1986, 'Selective birth', *Seminars in Perinatology* 10(1), 73–81.

Rhoads, G. G., Jackson, L. G., Schelesselman. S. *et al.*: 1989, 'The safety and efficacy of chorionic villus sampling for early prenatal diagnosis of cytogenetic abnormalities', *The New England Journal of Medicine* 320, 609–617.

Robie, G., Payne, G. Jr. and Morgan. M.: 1989, 'Selective delivery of an acardiac acephalic twin', *The New England Journal of Medicine* 320(8), 512–513.

Strong, C.: 1987, 'Ethical conflicts between mother and fetus', *Obstetrics and Gynecology Clinics in Perinatology* 14(2), 313–328.

U. S. Department of Health and Human Services, Office of Human Development Services: 1985, 'Child abuse and neglect prevention and treatment program', Final Rule, *Federal Register* 50(72), 14878–14892.

Wapner, R. J., Davis, G. H., Johnson, A. *et al.*: 1990, 'Selective reduction of multifetal pregnancies', *The Lancet* 335, 90–93.

Working Party on Children Conceived by *in vitro* fertilization, births in Great Britain resulting from assisted conception 1978–1987; 1990, British Medical Journal 300, 1229–1233.

JOHN C. HARVEY

THE FRAIL ELDERLY PERSON AND THOSE
SUFFERING FROM DEMENTIA

The world's population is graying. More people are living longer at the present time. This is occurring all over the world – not only in the highly industrialized countries, but also in the so-called developing world. The geriatric age group is the fastest growing segment in the population.

Individuals have been considered to be in the geriatric age group after the age of 65 years. Most retirement plans, pension payments (both private and governmental), and medical care plans for the elderly in every country have been geared to this age. Presently those individuals of 65 years are generally in very good health and vigorous. Some rethinking of this signpost is now taking place.

It is well known, however, that after 50 years of age, physiological age has no relationship to chronological age. We have all seen people who at age 65 years seem much, much older; and we've all seen the 95-year-old vigorous lady climbing about the Acropolis in comfortable running shoes and looking as though she were 42! Professor Bernice Neugarten of the University of Chicago, a long-time student of the sociology of aging did divide the geriatric population as a result of her studies into what she called the "young" old and the "old" old. Others have talked about the well elderly and the frail elderly. Generally the frail elderly do fall in the age group 75 years and upwards.

In the United States out of a population of some 250 million people, about 12% are in the geriatric population. This numbers some 30,800,000 individuals. This number is, of course, expected to grow in the next quarter century to about 20% of the population. Of this geriatric age group, quite surprising to most people, 95% are well elderly and 5% are frail elderly. Of the 5%, 2% are in nursing homes and another 3%, though severely impaired, are still living in the community.

To understand the implications of this reality, we must consider some basic concepts and facts. Studies of many investigators world wide (I use in particular the studies by Dr. Nathan Shock at the Gerontological Research Laboratories of the National Institutes of Health) show that in the normal aging process there is a decrease in organ reserve –

K.Wm. Wildes (ed.), Birth, Suffering and Death, 33–44.

"homeostenosis", a term coined by Dr. John Rowe, if you will. This is generally not relevant unless illness supervenes in the older individual. With loss of organ reserve, and loss of some function imposed by illness, the functioning of the geriatric patient is greatly restricted. We must remember that an individual is either well or ill. Illness is either acute and self-limited or chronic and progressive. An individual acutely ill either dies or recovers; that is, gets well and is restored to health and full vitality without any residual physiological alterations. An individual chronically ill has continued, and usually progressive, illness with the development to a greater or lesser degree of physiological deficits or handicaps. These physiological deficits or handicaps may be slight and without much effect upon the individual, or they may be severe and cause serious interference with the individual's ability to carry out his or her activities of daily living. If a person is so affected, he or she is considered disabled. The emotional attitude of the individual has a great influence upon that individual's ability to live to his or her fullest functional capacity.

The geriatric group is a hearty one. These people are survivors! They have survived the acute infections, trauma, and other physiological insults which are the causes of death in the younger age groups. The current geriatric population has survived the economic insult of the great world-wide depression in the 1930s, the physical and emotional drain of the Second World War, and the physical deprivations caused by the Cold War. The geriatric age group suffers not primarily from acute illness – though to be sure, that can occur – but from those illnesses that are chronic, long continuing, and causing physiological handicaps. Such diseases are rheumatoid arthritis, heart disease of various types, cerebrovascular disease and stroke, cancer, osteoporosis, diabetes, and Alzheimer's disease. These diseases are not primarily killers, but do cause severe physiological alterations which are long continuing and often progressive until the organ systems fail. Then death occurs. These physiological changes may prevent the individual from meeting his or her activities of daily living considered in the context of each one's sociological, economic, and educational circumstances. In this situation the individual is disabled. Now, as pointed out above, not all age-related physiological changes are caused by illness; some appear to be the natural outcome of the aging process. The unsteadiness of the elderly is an example of such a change. But functional reserves are present.

Thus it is important in the elderly to differentiate between acute and chronic illnesses, to determine the functional capacity of the individual, and to evaluate his or her ability to meet his or her needs of daily living within his or her sociological, economic, and educational environment. The determination of brain function or mental status is very important in this latter process.

If one studies various populations around the world, looking at the percentage of survivors of cohort groups through the years, one can see that more people are surviving over longer periods of time. If one looks at the tendency over the last eighty years as we have conquered the acute diarrheal diseases of infancy, the acute infectious processes such as rheumatic fever, small pox, tuberculosis, and poliomyelitis with development of preventive medicine measures such as immunization, the development of antibiotics, and better sanitary engineering – as we protect from and eliminate trauma of all kinds – we can see that there is a large survivor group over a long period of time, but then there is a sudden demise at the age of about 84.5 years. Fries at the Stanford University in California, looking at the possibility that death could occur by chance alone, has postulated that this point is the time for death as determined by the "genetic clock"; that is, the point of death if all disease and effects of trauma are eliminated from the human being. That this may well be true is suggested by the figures of continued life of both males and females after reaching the age of 65 years. In 1900 in the United States, if a male reached the age of 65 years, he had on the average eleven more years to live, a female slightly longer – thirteen years. In 1985, if a male lived to be 65 years of age, he could expect to live on the average fifteen more years, and a female seventeen more years. This slight lengthening of life after reaching the age of 65 years has been achieved in the last ninety years with all of their very tremendous advances in medicine, sanitary engineering, and sociological practices. The length of life has not really been extended appreciably at all. Thus the purpose of geriatric care is not to stretch the length of life like a rubber band to 120 or 150 years as some people wish, giving people Ponce de Leon's fountain of youth, but it is to make those years, allotted to man by the genetic clock, full, meaningful, and productive.

Yet this cannot be for all to live fully until the genetic clock runs out and death occurs rather quickly. Instead we see some in the geriatric population troubled most seriously with those chronic illnesses listed above which cause a deficit in their functional capacity. When social and economic status change these may cause such individuals with the decreased functional capacity to lose their ability to live independently.

Various assistances will be required, which may need to be provided by others – trained or untrained in health or personal care techniques. Now even lower primates (monkeys) are being trained for this activity in some medical centers.

The frail elderly individual, who has full brain capacity, can often, with such help, be maintained in his or her own residence, which psychologically and physically is the best situation. It has been shown over and over again when elderly individuals, even those with full brain capacity, are taken out of their usual and customary environments, they often become confused and may deteriorate physically in a very rapid fashion. When the frail elderly individual has some degree of brain failure (usually one of the dementias), the situation is more difficult. Often such individuals need constant, 24-hour surveillance and care. Thus they usually need placement in a nursing home or other appropriate, guarded, and supervised environment. Such movement, of course, hastens their deterioration.

The four great distinguishing symptoms of almost any illness (both physical and mental) in the frail elderly are best described by the four "I"s – incontinence, instability, immobility, and intellectual incapacitation. The first three are serious physical problems which coupled with the loss of organic reserve that the frail elderly usually exhibit (e.g., pulmonary disease, heart failure, renal impairment, and the like) create problems when such individuals remain in their own environment. Incontinence is usually not well-tolerated by family members and friends. It leads to isolation or institutionalization of the geriatric individual.

The instability (frequent falls) and the immobility from which many frail elderly suffer is not from the social standpoint as troublesome to others. These however do isolate the frail elderly and keep him or her at home or in the institution, but others do not find these two conditions intolerable.

Intellectual impairment or, as some British geriatricians term it, "brain failure", does create great problems for the frail elderly individual. This condition (dementia) is caused primarily (about 70% of the time) by two diseases – multiinfarct dementia and Alzheimer's disease. Another 10% of the dementias are associated with rather rare central nervous system diseases of the subcortical tissues, such as Huntington's Chorea, Parkinson's Disease, Jacob-Kruetzfeld Disease, and others even rarer. About 20% of the time intellectual impairment (brain failure or dementia) is caused by many diseases which, when properly diagnosed, may be correctable – e.g., hypothyroidism (myxedema), tuberculosis or fungal infection of the meninges (the lining of the brain), Vitamin B_6 or B_{12} deficiency and the like.

However, the two greatest causes for irreversible dementia are Alzheimer's disease and multiple microscopic areas of death of brain cells (infarcts) caused by multiple emboli coming from blood clots in the heart (a result of various heart diseases), by emboli breaking off from arteriosclerotic plaques in the carotid arteries (the two main arteries in the neck), or from actual disease of the small blood vessels in the brain. Dementia is not "just a process of aging". Dementia is the functional impairment resulting from disease and death of brain cells. It must be emphasized: it is always a disease, not a function of aging!

The various chronic diseases which may affect different organs of the body in different ways and the diseases of the brain listed above do not advance at equal rates. Thus one may be severely demented but have a rather strong body without significant physiological functional defects. We have all seen the elderly individual who is "as strong as an ox", but is very severely demented.

The instance of dementia, both the Alzheimer's variety and the multiinfarct variety appears to be increasing. Whether this is truly so (i.e., more cases are occurring) or that we are now making better diagnoses and not just ascribing brain failure to "old age" is unknown. Alzheimer's Disease accounted for the death of 100,000 Americans in 1988. Approximately one percent of the American population, or 2.5 million people are afflicted with this disease.

The courses of these two diseases do differ. With multiinfarct dementia progression is in step-down plateaus. With Alzheimer's disease progression is a steady deterioration. The patient with multiinfarct dementia retains his or her personality to a certain degree as well as the ability to carry out activities of daily living, though faulted on occasion. The person with multiinfarct dementia loses short-term memory but usually retains long-term memory.

In the early stages of both diseases, people are aware of their deficits in intellectual functioning. This engenders great frustration, anger, and often depression. It leads some patients to suicide – it leads others to ask for assisted suicide. As both the diseases progress, the burden increases for the caregiver. Often the stress and emotional drain on the caregiver cause greater anxiety and worry than for the patient.

Alzheimer's disease is one of the most horrifying to strike the elderly. It is also one of the most mysterious. Symptoms include severe loss of memory and personality changes which range from angry outbursts to withdrawal and depression. As it progresses there is a total loss of personality. The individual becomes a vacant automaton who knows no one, understands nothing, and appears to lose all learned information and motor functions. This full-blown picture is very stunning and frightening to family. There may be an hereditary tendency. Management of the patient is exceedingly burdensome, draining emotionally for the immediate caregivers, and expensive when given by third parties. The futility of the care since there is no cure, and the effort and energy expended by others for care leads many families to question whether it is worth it all. Some families consider the patient as dead, as a non-person but a living biological organism. This leads often to the family's speculation concerning the possibility of mercy killing as the only relief from intractable suffering.

The wife of an Alzheimer's patient in the early stages of the disease once said jokingly that her husband was so happy because he met a new woman every morning – namely his wife! However, progression of Alzheimer's disease can be rapid,and death may occur within one or two years. On the other hand, the course of the illness can be painfully slow. The usual length of life after the diagnosis has been made is about five to seven years, though it may be somewhat longer. The duration of life after the development of multiinfarct dementia varies anywhere from five to twenty years, though shorter periods of time than twenty years are more common. Usually death is from some vascular event such as cerebral hemorrhage or intercurrent infections.

Demographically speaking, the aging of the population refers to the increasing proportion of older people rather than a spectacular gain in absolute numbers.[1] At the turn of the century, the United States was a demographically youthful country. Only about 4% of the total population was 65 years or over. By 1950, the United States could be considered to be a "mature" country with an older population of 8.1%. In 1980, the population over age 65 years was 11.3%. The United States, however, is far from being the "oldest" of the developed countries. Sweden, Norway, Denmark, the United Kingdom, and West Germany each have had over 15% of their populations age 65 and over in 1988. It is important to realize that changes in the proportion of the elderly, unlike changes in absolute numbers, are affected by a variations in the numbers of people in other age categories. Basically, an increase in the proportion of the population age 65 years and over is due more to declining fertility than to lower death rates. The drop in fertility over the last 15 to 20 years in the United States reduces the proportion of young persons and thus increases the proportion of adults and older persons in the population. As time goes on, because of these changes in relative numbers of persons, those age 85 years and over will constitute 1 in 4 of all elderly persons. Increasing numbers of older persons have increased demands for the goods and services that the aged are prone to consume. Increasing proportions of elderly point to the difficulties that could be encountered in absorbing the cost of meeting this escalating demand. Age-dependency ratios are one way of estimating society's capacity to maintain the quality of life of older persons. In 1985 there were about 19 persons of retirement age for every 100 working persons. This ratio is projected to increase to 21 by the year 2000, and by 2050 the age-dependency ratio will more than double from its 1985 level to 38. This increase implies an increasing financial burden on workers in the next century under the current system.

The older population, especially the "old" old, is predominantly female. Six out of every 10 older Americans are women. This sex imbalance in the older population, of course, reflects higher male mortality. Sex differentials in survivorship rates have great importance, because older men and women have quite different social and economic resources available. In general, older women have fewer financial assets, and because they typically outlive their spouses, are more dependent on adult children and formal health services (including nursing homes) to meet their needs.

The "oldest" old, those 85 years of age and over, are the fastest growing age group within our entire population. While the older population as a whole increased 11% between 1980 and 1985 in the United States, the number of those 85 years of age and over increased by 20%. By the year 2000, the number of people age 65 years and older is expected to increase by an additional 22%, while the number of "oldest" old is likely to increase by an astounding 82%. There is an unequal geographic distribution of the older individuals in the United States. Over one-third of all older persons in the United States live in the South, which is proportional to that region's total population share. The Northeast and the Midwest have more aged relative to total population. The West has less than one-fifth of its population in the older age groups, which is less than its share of total population. The state of Florida has the largest proportion of elderly with 17.7% of its population 65 years or over in 1986.

The risk of functional disability increases rapidly after the age of 65 years. Nearly half of those individuals age 85 years and over have some difficulty performing at least one of the seven activities of daily living. It is to be emphasized again that although very few older people not in institutions are disease free, a majority manifest little, if any, functional incapacitation. This is contrary to the popular stereotypes. Frailty is not synonymous with old age. It is important to realize also that disability is more reversible than previously thought possible.

After health, economic and social resources make the greatest difference in the quality of daily life for older people. Older people have less cash income than younger people, and spend relatively more of their income on food, housing, and health care. Most older women are widows, and 51% of women 75 years of age and over have lived alone their whole lives. There is significant variation between wealth and poverty in the income distribution of the elderly. Personal income usually drops by one-third to one-half with retirement. With that cut, many older persons encounter poverty for the first time in their lives. In 1986 in the United States, 1 in 8, or 12%, of the elderly had incomes below the poverty level. Poverty rates increase with age, even among the elderly. In 1986, almost 1 in 5 of the elderly over age 85 years lived below the poverty level. Poverty rates are also higher for elderly women than men. Older people's financial status depends a great deal on where their money comes from. Most rely upon a mix of sources – Social Security benefits, pensions (both public and private), and income from savings and investments. Social Security in the United States is by far the most important of these.

The expenditure for health care for the elderly is increasing dramatically. In 1980 one-third of the health care dollar in the United States was spent on about 11% of the population, the elderly; whereas in 2020, it will be about one-half of the health care dollar that will be spent on the 20% of the elderly in the population. It is interesting to note that of the expenditures by Medicare, one-third of these are spent in the last two months of life. This has led many to question these expenditures as being futile.

There are many challenges of long-term care. By far the most pervasive and the most costly problem of older individuals is personal care. At $20,000 per year for home care, and about $36,000 per year for nursing home care, even a relatively brief episode of long-term care can bankrupt most older families, whose median income in 1986 was $19,922. Compounding the cost problems of long-term care is a fragmented approach to the delivery of personal care services. Older persons needing help in the United States must travel through a maze of independent applications for Medicaid, Social Security insurance, Title XX and Title III programs. Viewed from a policy perspective, this piecemeal approach to the delivery of community long-term care services encourages admissions to institutions, the majority of which ultimately are paid for by Medicare. To test innovative strategies for reducing rates of unnecessary nursing home use and public expenditures for long-term care, as well as improving the quality of life for the frail elderly, the federal government has funded at least 16 demonstration projects since 1970. Cost savings, as measured in terms of aggregate expenditures for long-term care, have been trivial in most of these experimental programs.

The debate on expanded home-care services will not be decided on the basis of research. Ultimately the public policy agenda must come to grips with the value basis by which scarce federal resources are allocated to support the long-term well-being and satisfaction of older citizens. In a pluralistic society such as America, value-based conflicts can be resolved only through the workings of the political process. The ongoing debate on expanded long-term care benefits will be particularly difficult to resolve because it will be played out in the context of increasing concern over the federal deficit. As the four generation family becomes more prevalent, the awareness of the issue will undoubtedly increase. Already one survey estimates that 60% of the adults in the United States have had first hand experience dealing with the emotional and financial costs of long-term care. While there is widespread support for the general notion that we have a collective obligation to provide for those who previously con- tributed to the growth and development of our country, at issue today, however, is the extent of this commitment. The competition among various groups for federal program dollars is partly due to cutbacks in domestic spending during the Reagan administration. There is, nonethe- less, a growing perception that improved benefits for older persons have come at the expense of diminished well-being for children and middle- aged workers, raising the issue of intergenerational inequity. Central to the intergenerational equity debate are Social Security taxes. Contrary to popular misconception, payroll deductions are not deposited into individual accounts for the eventual retirement of the contributing workers. Our Social Security system is not an annuity system, but a program of direct structured intergenerational transfers. Most of the $215 billion paid by about 122 million workers in 1986 went to provide monthly benefits to 23 million retirees and 2.5 million disabled persons.

In the early 1980s, the future viability of the Social Security system was the center of national debate. Changes were made and a scheduled increase in payroll deductions and gradual increase in the full benefit retirement age from 65 to age 67 by 2026 were worked out to save the Social Security system. The direct effect of these changes will be to increase the financial burden on workers in the short run and to delay their claim on retirement benefits in the long run. The intergenerational equity is more than a strict accounting of costs and benefits to different age groups. It presumes competition and forecasts conflict. Inherent in this framework are the questionable assumptions that total federal revenues are fixed and that increased spending for one group can only come at the expense of the needs of other groups. The intergenerational equity argument is most likely to come up in the next decade with respect to the financing of long-term care for the elderly. The debate will likely center on ways to underwrite the cost of expanded long-term care under either Medicare or Medicaid.

The ethical issues which arise in consideration of the frail elderly person and those suffering from dementia may be considered under two general headings: Ethical issues associated with the individual frail or demented person and ethical issues involving the society at large of which the frail or demented person is a part. I have hinted at some of these in the various paragraphs above. Other papers in this volume will deal with some of these ethical issues more specifically and in greater detail (e.g., Bole; O'Rourke; Bader; Schotsmans).

The frail elderly person and the individual with early dementia (of either major variety –   multi-infarct or Alzheimer's) often dislikes the diminishment of human dignity which is imposed by the illness and its subsequent effect upon functional capacity. An individual who must go into diapers because of urinary and fecal incontinence is greatly concerned about dignity. The person with early dementia often expresses concern for the results of the ongoing process. The individual feels that progressive diminution of mental capacity – the ever relentless progressive brain failure – is a personal affront to dignity (Ashley; Autiero; Schotsmans, this volume). Many individuals in their despair for the future express wishes to avoid this suffering by talking of suicide, assisted suicide, or euthanasia. Family members fully informed of the condition of the frail or demented individual and the prognosis truly wish for their loved ones an avoidance of this diminution of dignity and its concomitant suffering. Family members may speak of euthanasia as an alternative to the expected and inevitable diminution of dignity. The financial burdens which the illness of the frail elderly and demented persons have imposed upon the patient, the spouse, or other family members may lead to physical impoverishment (Bole, this volume). Such physical impoverishment may result in loss of accustomed life style, loss of companions and friends, poor housing, and hunger. It also may lead to spiritual impoverishment, causing disenchantment, despair, and depression. The necessary medical treatment may be foregone by the patient to avoid the financial burdens in favor of expenditures for activities considered of greater value by the patient such as the spouse's well-being after his death, family members need for financial assistance for education or housing, etc (Bole, this volume). This often leads to familial guilt and quarreling. As illness progresses decisions regarding use of high technological procedures in the terminal stages of the illness can lead to disruption of family harmony when differences of opinion arise over issues of autonomy, substituted judgement, interpretation of advanced directives, termination of medical treatment and the like (Bader; Schotsmans; Paris; Bole; O'Rourke; this volume).

For society at large the ethical issues concerning the frail elderly individual and the person with dementia revolve around the issues of distributive justice. How much claim do the geriatric patients have for society's resources for health care? The rapid and ever rising costs for wages of health care workers, for equipment and facilities for long-term care given either at home or in the institutional setting, and for terminal care of individuals often rendered in the intensive care units of acute hospitals (the most expensive of all the levels of care) and almost always perceived as ineffective and even futile, leads the society to express the bias of ageism – the third and newest general social bias after racism and sexism. These facts call for an exploration of the ethical issues involved in distributive justice.

Ethical issues arise for the individuals in society who form the cadre of heath care givers. Doctors, nurses, allied health-care workers, and others are faced often with conflictual situations in their work over ethical issues of autonomy verses beneficence, of virtuous behavior in the face of demands of patients and families incompatible with the given health-care giver's moral stance, and issues in which utilitarian principles clash with deontological ones.

The unprecedented increase in the number of older people and the rapidity of the growth of their share in total population in almost every country as well as the United States is a new social phenomenon, offering both problems and opportunities. These create many ethical problems, which have to be faced courageously and yet realistically.

NOTE

[1] Much of the information in this and subsequent paragraphs comes from the studies of Professor Beth Soldo.

BIBLIOGRAPHY

AMA Council on Scientific Affairs: 1990, 'Societal ethics and other factors affecting health care for the elderly', *Archieves of Internal Medicine*, 150, 1184–1189.

Brock, Dan W.: 1989, 'Justice, health care, and the elderly', *Philosophy and Public Affairs*, 18, 297–312.

Brocklehurst, J. C. (ed.): 1990, 'Management of urinary incontinence in the community', *Gerontology, International Journal of Experimental and Clinical Gerontology*, 36, supplement 2.

Callahan, Daniel: 1973, *The Tyranny of Survival*. MacMillan, New York.

Cassel, C. K.: 1988, 'Health care for an aging America', *Bulletin of the Park Ridge Center*, September/October, Park Ridge Center, Chicago.

Christiansen, Drew: 1974, 'Diginity in aging', *Hastings Center Report*, February, 6–8.

Cohn, V.: 1989, 'When painful days are numbered', *Washington Post*, July 25.

Coni, N., Davison, W., & Webster, S.: 1980, *Lecture Notes on Geriatrics*, 2nd edition, Blackwell, Oxford.

Feder, J.: 1990, 'Health care of the disadvantaged: The elderly', *Journal of Health, Policy, and Law*, 259–269.

Klein, L., German, P. S. & Levine, D.: 'Adverse drug reactions among the elderly: A reassessment', *Journal of the American Geriatrics Society*, 29, 525–530.

Lamm, R. D.: 1989, 'Critical decisions in medical care: Birth to death', *Southern Medical Journal*, 822–824.

Otten, A. L.: 1988, 'The Geratrician needs special skills, patience and a sense of humor', *Wall Street Journal*, January 25.

Perlin, E.: 1990, 'Jewish medical ethics and the care of the elderly', *Pharos*, Summer, 2–5.

Shanas, E. *et al.*: 1968, *Old People in Three Industrial Societies*, Atherton, New York.

Soldo, B. J. and Agree, E. M.: 1988, 'America's elderly', *Population Bulletin*, 43, No. 3. Population Reference Bureau, Inc., Washington, DC.

EDWIN CASSEM S.J.

THE HIV INFECTION

The acquired immunodeficiency syndrome (AIDS) can well be considered the greatest health crisis in the twentieth century. This paper
reviews the epidemiology, cause, clinical course, and prevention and
treatment of the disease.

I. THE EPIDEMIOLOGY OF AIDS (OSMOND, 1990)

By July, 1990, 206, 217 cases of AIDS had been reported to the World
Health Organization. The true number is unknown, but the WHO
estimated that it was 250,000 by the end of 1988. Of the cases reported to
the WHO 137,385 came from the United States. More than 5 million
persons worldwide are believed to be asymptomatic carriers of HIV, the
retrovirus that causes AIDS. The best current U.S. estimate is more than
one million infections, (*MMWR 1990; 39: 110–119, JAMA, 3/16/90*)
ranging between 0.5 and 3 million. Eight to ten million people worldwide
are infected with the virus, half of them in Africa. Data from prospective
studies of HIV-seropositive individuals suggest that essentially all of
these persons will become afflicted by AIDS, although the median time
from infection to getting AIDS is now about 10 years. The U.S. Public
Health Service extrapolated infection trends to estimate that a cumulative
total of 480,000 cases will occur by the end of 1993, with up to 340,000
AIDS-related deaths.

There are basically three patterns of case reporting throughout the
world which represent two distinct forms of the disease. The first pattern,
found in North and South America, Western Europe, Scandinavia,
Australia, and New Zealand, is associated with infection by one form of
the virus, HIV-1, which causes most of the cases of AIDS worldwide.
Ninety percent of these cases have occurred in homosexuals and IV drug
abusers. A second form of the virus, HIV-2, causes a second pattern of
infection and occurs in Africa, the Caribbean and some areas of South
America. The primary mode of transmission for this virus appears to be
heterosexual and the number of cases is equal between males and

45

K.Wm. Wildes (ed.), Birth, Suffering and Death, 45–65.
© 1992 *Kluwer Academic Publishers. Printed in the Netherlands.*

females. For that reason, because of the high percentage of females infected, the rate of perinatal infection is extremely high. A third pattern occurs in Eastern Europe, North Africa, the Middle East, Asia and the Pacific (except for Australia and New Zealand), where there are either few AIDS cases or defective reporting. There is reason to believe, for example, that the disease in the Soviet Union is not only frequent but has actually been spread by hospitals and clinics because of the unavailability of disposable needles and syringes and the impossibility of implementing adequate precautions against the virus.

The distribution of AIDS cases in the United States, where there were only two states with more than 5,000 cases reported as of 1989, New York and California, reveals a lesson about this disease. AIDS is a disease of large cities. New York, San Francisco, and Los Angeles are cities in the United States with a heavy infection rate with HIV-1. An understanding of the makeup of the patient population is also instructive. In San Francisco, for example, the proportion of homosexuals with the disease to IV drug abusers is 90 to 10, whereas in New York the proportion is closer to 50/50. For this reason, epidemiologists are quite hopeful about progress being made in the control of the disease in San Francisco but quite pessimistic about the control of the disease in New York City, where the prevalence rate of HIV infection is 10 times higher than in the U.S. as a whole.

Based on United States public health projections of 1988, it is estimated that by the end of 1992 there will be in the U.S. 365,000 cumulative cases, 263,000 cumulative deaths, 80,000 cases diagnosed during 1992, 66,000 deaths during 1992, and 172,000 patients in 1992 requiring medical care. The cost range for 1992 alone is estimated to range between 5 and 13 billion dollars.

Four groups account for most of the HIV-1 cases in the first pattern of infection (percentages differ from country to country; those given are for the United States): homosexual or bisexual men (73 %); heterosexual men or women who are intravenous drug users (17 %); recipients of transfusions, all of whom received transfusions before blood testing became possible in 1983 (2 %); and hemophiliacs (1 %). Surveillance data from San Francisco indicate that the seroconversion rates in homosexual and bisexual men have leveled off and are decreasing. This trend should continue in other urban centers. Heterosexual transmission has accounted for about 4 % of adult cases for the past five years, but is increasing. As the epidemic continues to escalate among IV drug users, heterosexual transmission and infection rates in women will increase. Currently HIV-1 infection is far more common in men than in women. However, by 1991 HIV/AIDS can be expected to become one of the five leading causes of death in women of reproductive age (Chu *et al.*, 1990).

By the end of 1988, 1,346 cases had been reported in children younger than 13 years. Although some were hemophiliac children, 75 % were infected *in utero* by a mother who was herself an IV drug user or was infected by one. HIV-1 can be transmitted by breast feeding as well. As of July 1989 children represented fewer than 2 % of all of the cases of AIDS in the United States.

In the U.S., the incidence of AIDS is three times higher in blacks and Hispanics than in whites. Most of the black and Hispanic AIDS patients have a history of intravenous drug abuse, have acquired the disease from heterosexual contact with someone at high risk for acquiring AIDS, or are children.

It became possible to screen donated blood and plasma for antibody to HIV in April of 1985. In addition, donor screening on the basis of history had made it possible to exclude high risk donors prior to this, and, finally, heat treatment of clotting factor concentrates has been added so that the safety of the blood supply in the U.S. and Europe is essentially assured. It is possible that a unit of blood that had been tested negative by current enzyme-linked immunosorbent assays (ELISA) could contain and transmit HIV. The likelihood that infection will be transmitted in this fashion is estimated to be, at its upper limit, between 1 in 100,000 and 1 in 1 million per unit of blood. (Seventy percent of the entire hemophiliac population in the United States are now infected with HIV.) If an infected donor unit of blood is used, the risk of the recipient incurring HIV infection is at least 66 %. If AIDS develops in such a blood donor within 23 months of donation, all recipients of the donor's blood will become infected. Likewise, if one recipient of blood from a particular donor is infected, all recipients will be infected.

Clearly the most worrisome sub-population with AIDS is the IV drug-abusing population, in which the epidemic is still worsening. A recent study from the New York City area indicated that 5 out of 6 of these patients have, in addition to AIDS, syphilis, gonorrhea, and/or hepatitis. Twenty-five percent of them were homeless and 80 % were unemployed. Only 15 % of IV drug abusers seek treatment for addiction. As yet, educational methods and distribution of clean needles to IV drug abusers have not been demonstrated to be effective, but are currently under investigation. The number of IV drug users in the U.S. is currently estimated to be 750,000.

II. THE NATURE OF THE DISEASE: THE CULPRIT, THE RETROVIRUS

The nomenclature of the virus has at times been confusing. One of the discoverers of the virus, Luc Montagnier, of the Pasteur Institute of Paris, first named the virus the lymphadenopathy virus (LAV). Robert Gallo, one of the co-discoverers in the United States, referred to it as human T-cell lymphotropic virus, type III (HTLV-III). It has also been referred to as AIDS-related virus (ARV). By consensus, all now refer to the virus as human immunodeficiency virus (HIV). Because there are two types, this virus is known as HIV-1. The second type of retrovirus, which is much more similar in genetic form to the simian immunodeficiency virus (SIV), and is present chiefly in West Africa, is referred to as HIV-2. It was originally also referred to as HTLV-IV.

The agent which transmits the disease has been classified as a retrovirus. The discovery of its exact structure and detailed genetic code is certainly among the most dramatic scientific achievements of the 20th century. The particle itself is known as a virion. As shown in Fig. 1, it can be described as a spherical particle with protruding knob-like particles, referred to as gp120. (The numbers on the labels refer to the molecular weight of the protein, in this case 120,000 daltons.) Thus, the protein which anchors gp120 to the lipid bilayer surface of the virion, gp41, is a protein with a molecular weight of 41 kilodaltons. The virus's core appears to be surrounded by another protein, called p24. Within the core, along with the RNA carrying the virus's genetic information, are two enzymes, DNA-polymerase and ribonuclease, which together are often called reverse transcriptase. The combination of these enzymes enables the virus to make DNA corresponding to the RNA. It is for this reason that the virus is called a retrovirus, i.e., the genetic process, compared to human replication, goes "backward". In ordinary cells, DNA makes RNA in order to transmit itself. The retrovirus produces DNA from RNA.

The virion particles attack human T4 lymphocytes. In the body's immune system, which could be thought of as a naval defense fleet against disease, the T4 cell, sometimes known as a helper T cell, could be viewed as the flagship of the defense. The virus, in sinking these ships, deals eventually an irreversible blow to the body's ability to reject the infection.

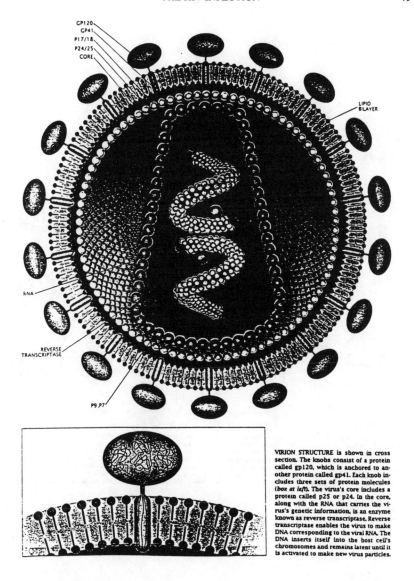

VIRION STRUCTURE is shown in cross section. The knobs consist of a protein called gp120, which is anchored to another protein called gp41. Each knob includes three sets of protein molecules (box at left). The virus's core includes a protein called p25 or p24. In the core, along with the RNA that carries the virus's genetic information, is an enzyme known as reverse transcriptase. Reverse transcriptase enables the virus to make DNA corresponding to the viral RNA. The DNA inserts itself into the host cell's chromosomes and remains latent until it is activated to make new virus particles.

Fig. 1. Gallo RC, Montagnier L. AIDS in 1988. In *Scientific American* (vol. 259, no. 4), 41–47 (p. 43).

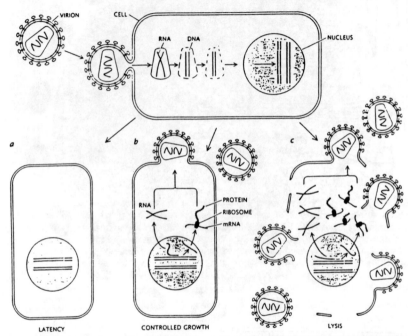

Fig. 2. Haseltine WA, Wong-Staal F. The molecular biology of the AIDS virus. In *Scientific American* (vol. 259, no. 4), 52–62 (p. 54).

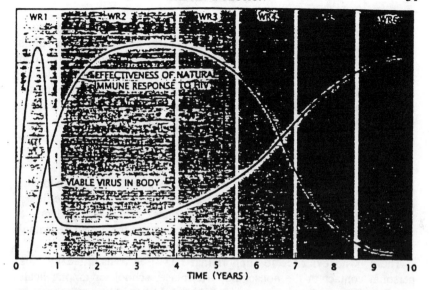

BALANCE OF POWER between HIV (*black curve*) and the immune system (*red curve*) shifts during the course of the infection, according to a model proposed by the authors. The amount of HIV in the body soars in the first days of infection, but once the immune system "kicks in," it initially operates normally and reduces the amount of virus. The immune system remains in good control of the virus for several years, but HIV gains ground slowly. At some point the T4 cells that orchestrate the immune response become so depleted that the balance of power switches. HIV then replicates wildly, killing the remaining T4 cells and hence any vestiges of immune defense.

Fig. 3. Redfield RR, Burke DS. HIV infection: The clinical picture. In *Scientific American* (vol. 259, no. 4), 90–98 (p. 97).

The process of infection occurs when the gp120 knobs attach themselves to a receptor on the T4 cell known as CD4 (Fig. 2). Through this attachment the core of the virion with its RNA is introduced into the cell. Once within the cell, reverse transcriptase makes first one strand of DNA from RNA, then, after destroying the second strand of RNA a second strand of DNA is made and these two strands of viral DNA are then introduced into the nucleus of the T cell, where they infiltrate the genetic DNA of the cell and essentially take command of the replicating machinery of the T cell. From this point the T cell may go into a stage of latency, simply carrying around the lethal code within the cell but not producing virions. Another T cell may produce controlled growth in which virions are produced by the genetic machinery and periodically eliminated into the blood stream where they attach themselves to other T cells and take command of the nucleic genetic machinery in a similar fashion. There are times when several infected T cells form a conglomerate syncytial cell, which at some point will disintegrate, releasing multiple virions into the circulation. It is also possible for the virion to infect monocytes and macrophage cells and it is thought that infected macrophages carry the HIV infection into the brain.

III. WHAT IS THE NATURE OF THE CLINICAL DISEASE?

Basically, one finds persons in one of three categories: asymptomatic patients carrying HIV infection, infected patients with an immune illness, and infected patients with a neurologic illness. There are patients, of course, who overlap in the latter two categories and have both neurologic and immunologic manifestations of the illness.

There is no evidence to support that HIV-1 is transmitted by close personal contact in the household, workplace, school, or among health care workers who have no exposure to blood. Insects, like mosquitoes, are shown not to transmit HIV-1 infection. Hence, persons who are afraid that the virus may be transmitted by food or water, coughing, or sneezing should be reassured that this has not been demonstrated to be the case.

Although most of the persons infected with HIV initially show no signs and feel completely well, the initial infection can actually produce symptoms. Some people will report a fever, rash, flu-like symptoms, and occasionally symptoms of meningitis (headache, photophobia, stiff neck). This is thought likely to occur if there was a rapid replication and release of virus in the blood stream at the time of seroconversion. Yet in most patients their immune system contains the viral infection and there are no manifestations of disease.

The incubation after seroconversion is much longer than originally thought, and appears to have a median duration of 9 to 10 years.

One way to view the disease progression is to think of it in parallel with loss of the body's own ability to contain the virus. Figures 3 and 4 show the Walter-Reed stages of HIV infection. In effect, the more T4 helper cells are infected, the more vulnerable the individual becomes. Among its other functions, this helper T cell is the cell which recognizes foreign cells (antigens) and then mobilizes the rest of the immune "fleet" to attack the invaders.

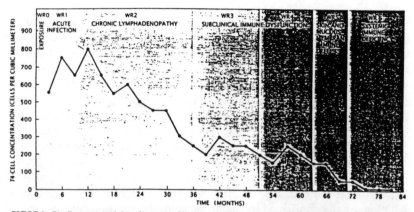

DECLINE in T4-cell count (rounded to the nearest 50) was tracked in the blood of a young man whose disease followed a typical course. About three months after sexual exposure to HIV the patient tested positive for the virus; his T4-cell count dropped and then rebounded, presumably because his immune system temporarily controlled the infection. He developed chronic lymphadenopathy at nine months and, at 51 months, after a long, slow decline in his T4-cell count (by 36 months it was chronically below 400), exhibited chronic, subtle abnormalities of delayed hypersensitivity. He displayed persistent anergy (the complete absence of delayed hypersensitivity) at 63 months but had no overt symptoms of infection until about 68 months, when he developed thrush and oral hairy leukoplakia, a tongue infection. Less than a year later he was besieged by opportunistic infections, including cytomegalovirus infection, which made him blind. He died at 83 months.

Fig. 4. Redfield RR, Burke DS. HIV infection: The clinical picture. In *Scientific American* (vol. 259, no. 4), 90–98 (p. 94).

Basically, the B (killer) lymphocytes, which represent the majority of the rest of the fleet, multiply and produce specific antibodies which bind to infected cells, enabling the body to then destroy infected cells. The steady decline of helper T cells makes it increasingly difficult for the patient's immune system to reject infection. One of the earliest signs, marking stage 2 of the 6 stages of the illness, is the swelling of lymph nodes, discovered by the patient typically in the neck, groins and axillae. With a normal T4 cell count being 800 or more, stage 3 is defined when the T4 cell population drops to 400 cells per cubic millimeter of blood. At this point a patient, when tested by four special skin tests, usually fails to mobilize a defense in three out of four. The patient then passes into stage 5 when he fails completely to respond to the skin tests or when a fungal infection called thrush produces white spots in the mouth. These are often sore and a source of discomfort to the patient. Thrush can also be detected by the formation of small ulcerated areas in the mouth, on the tongue or on other sites of the mucous membranes lining the oral cavity. As stage 5 progresses, the truly serious viral and fungal infections begin to occur. One of the commonest is chronic infection with Candida, the fungus that causes thrush, which may begin to spread throughout areas, such as the vagina. Herpes simplex, which produces painful sores around the mouth, on the skin, and around the anus and genital area, begins to persist and cause a great deal of discomfort for the patient. Another stage 5 complication is called hairy leukoplakia, an infection manifested by fuzzy white spots on the tongue that cannot be rubbed off. The cause for these is not clear. Within a year or two after entering stage 5, patients go on to develop chronic or disseminated opportunistic infections. When these occur, immune competence has reached a severely low level. The duration of Stages 2 to 5 is quite variable, but once symptoms develop, roughly half of those infected will acquire AIDS by the end of two years.

It is usually in stage 6 that the patient receives a definite diagnosis of AIDS; that is the end stage of HIV infection. However, the diagnosis of AIDS is usually confirmed by the presence of the severe forms of some of these infections, such as candidiasis of the esophagus, lungs, bronchi or trachea; cryptococcosis; cryptospiridiosis with diarrhea persisting for more than one month; cytomegalovirus (CMV) disease of an organ other than the liver, spleen, or lymph nodes in a patient older than one month; herpes simplex infection causing a mucocutaneous ulcer that persists longer than one month of HSV infection causing bronchitis, pneumonitis or esophagitis for any duration; Kaposi's sarcoma in a patient younger than 60 years; lymphoma of the brain; Mycobacterium avium complex disease, disseminated (most commonly manifested as severe diarrhea); Pneumocystis carinii pneumonia; progressive multifocal leukoencephalopathy, a severe rapidly progressive dementing viral infection of the brain; toxoplasmosis of the brain in a patient older than one month. In such patients, even if the laboratory tests for HIV infection gave inconclusive results, the diagnosis of AIDS would be made. If the diagnosis of HIV is confirmed, then a diagnosis of AIDS is made under the conditions described in Table 1. Notable in the Table are the presence of HIV encephalopathy (II.A.4) and HIV wasting syndrome (II.A.5), conditions in which no additional viral or bacterial infection may be discovered, but in the former case the patient is becoming slowly demented, and in the latter case the patient is progressively losing weight and is unable, in spite of vigorous feeding, to prevent a state that looks like progressive malnutrition and starvation.

TABLE 1

CDC Surveillance Case Definition for AIDS

I. HIV Status of Patient Is Unknown or Inconclusive

If laboratory tests for HIV infection were not performed or gave inconclusive results and the patient had no other cause of immunodeficiency listed in IA (see below), a definitive diagnosis of any disease listed in IB (see below) indicates AIDS.

A. *Causes of immunodeficiency that disqualify a disease as an indication of AIDS in the absence of laboratory evidence of HIV infection*

1. The use of high-dose or long-term systemic corticosteroid therapy or other immunosuppressive/cytotoxic therapy within three months before the onset of the indicator disease.

2. A diagnosis of any of the following diseases within three months after diagnosis of the indicator disease: Hodgkin's disease, non-Hodgkin's lymphoma (other than primary brain lymphoma), lymphocytic leukemia, multiple myeloma, any other cancer of lymphoreticular or histiocytic tissue, or angioimmunoblastic lymphadenopathy.

3. A genetic (congenital) immunodeficiency syndrome or an acquired immunodeficiency syndrome that is atypical of HIV infection, such as one involving hypogammaglobulinemia.

B. *Diseases that indicate AIDS (requires definitive diagnosis)*

1. Candidiasis of the esophagus, trachea, bronchi, or lungs.

2. Cryptococcosis, extrapulmonary.

3. Cryptosporidiosis with diarrhea persisting for more than one month.

4. Cytomegalovirus disease of an organ other than the liver, spleen, or lymph nodes in a patient older than one month.

5. Herpes simplex virus infection causing a mucocutaneous ulcer that persists longer than one month; or herpes simplex virus infection causing bronchitis, pneumonitis, or esophagitis for any duration in a patient older than one month.

6. Kaposi's sarcoma in a patient younger than 60 years.

7. Lymphoid interstitial pneumonia or pulmonary lymphoid hyperplasia (LIP/PLH complex) in a patient younger than 13 years.

8. Lymphoma of the brain (primary) affecting a patient younger than 60 years.

9. *Mycobacterium avium* complex or *M. kansasii* disease, disseminated (at a site other than or in addition to the lungs, skin, or cervical or hilar lymph nodes).

10. *Pneumocystis carinii* pneumonia.

11. Progressive multifocal leukoencephalopathy.

12. Toxoplasmosis of the brain in a patient older than one month.

II. Patient Is HIV Positive

Regardless of the presence of other causes of immunodeficiency (see IA, above), in the presence of laboratory evidence of HIV infection, any disease listed in IB (see above) or in IIA or IIB (see below) indicates a diagnosis of AIDS.

A. *Diseases that indicate AIDS (requires definitive diagnosis)*

1. Bacterial infections, multiple or recurrent (any combination of at least two within a two- to four-year period), of the following types in a patient younger than 13 years: septicemia, pneumonia, meningitis, bone or joint infection, or abscess of an internal organ or body cavity (excluding otitis media or superficial skin or mucosal abscesses) caused by *Hemophilus, Streptococcus* (including pneumococcus), or other pyogenic bacteria.

2. Coccidioidomycosis, disseminated (at a site other than or in addition to the lungs or cervical or hilar lymph nodes).

3. Histoplasmosis, disseminated (at a site other than or in addition to the lungs or cervical or hilar lymph nodes).

4. HIV encephalopathy.

5. HIV wasting syndrome.

6. Isosporiasis with diarrhea persisting for more than one month.

7. Kaposi's sarcoma at any age.

8. Lymphoma of the brain (primary) at any age.

9. *M. tuberculosis* disease, extrapulmonary (involving at least one site outside the lungs, regardless of whether there is concurrent pulmonary involvement).

10. Mycobacterial disease caused by mycobacteria other than *M. tuberculosis*, disseminated (at a site other than or in addition to the lungs, skin, or cervical or hilar lymph nodes).

11. Non-Hodgkin's lymphoma of B cell or unknown immunologic phenotype and the following histologic types: small noncleaved lymphoma (Burkitt's or non-Burkitt's) or immunoblastic sarcoma.

12. *Salmonella* (nontyphoidal) septicemia, recurrent.

B. *Diseases that indicate AIDS (presumptive diagnosis)*

1. Candidiasis of the esophagus.

2. Cytomegalovirus retinitis, with loss of vision.

3. Kaposi's sarcoma.

4. Lymphoid interstitial pneumonia or pulmonary lymphoid hyperplasia (LIP/PLH complex) in a patient younger than 13 years.

5. Mycobacterial disease (acid-fast bacilli with species not identified by culture), disseminated (involving at least one site other than or in addition to the lungs, skin, or cervical or hilar lymph nodes).

6. *P. carinii* pneumonia.

7. Toxoplasmosis of the brain in a patient older than one month.

III. Patient Is HIV Negative

With laboratory test results negative for HIV infection, a diagnosis of AIDS for surveillance purposes is ruled out unless

A. All the other causes of immunodeficiency listed in IA (see above) are excluded; *and*

B. The patient has had either of the following:

1. *P. carinii* pneumonia diagnosed by a definitive method.

2. A definitive diagnosis of any of the other diseases indicative of AIDS listed in IB (see above) and a CD4+ helper-inducer T cell count of less than 400/mm³.

Note: Reference 1 provides a complete commentary and explanation of these criteria, including criteria for diagnosis.

Rubin RH. Acquired immunodeficiency syndrome. In: Rubenstein E, Federman DD, eds. *Scientific American Medicine* 7.XI.1–20, New York: Scientific American, 1989 (p. 2).

THE BRAIN IN AIDS

The central nervous system manifestations of HIV-1 infection are multiple. As was mentioned, there may be a mild syndrome of aseptic meningitis early in the course of the illness. Between 5 and 10 % of the patients experience this infection, associated with HIV seroconversion. The symptoms are fever, headache, occasional photophobia, a feeling of general malaise, and occasionally some difficulty with the facial muscles and hearing. It is short-lived, although the symptoms may be quite distressing during the brief period when the disease is present.

The milder forms of the cognitive changes occur while the patient is still in stages 3 and 4 of the disease. The more severe forms of the dementia ordinarily occur when immune function falls in what would ordinarily be known as stage 5 or 6 disease. It can be the case, as was noted, that the sole manifestation of HIV infection is a slow, progressive, dementing illness.

There is another severe neurologic complication of AIDS known as vacuolar myelopathy, which occurs in 11 to 22 % of AIDS patients. It commonly accompanies dementia and is manifested by a progressive spastic weakness of the legs with unsteady gait, weakness, and loss of bowel and bladder control. This may progress to paralysis of a limb and is extremely debilitating.

The HIV encephalopathy, also known as subacute encephalitis, and AIDS dementia, is a complex of cognitive, motor, behavioral, and affective abnormalities. There are highly variable presentations and the most sensitive point for the diagnostician becomes when to make this diagnosis, which is so potentially devastating for the patient. Thus, the early manifestations will almost always include memory loss, impaired concentration, some slowing of both motor and cognitive function, comprehension difficulties, and some mild conceptual confusion. Apathy, depressive mood, a sense of agitation or even some psychotic features, like hallucinations or paranoid delusions, may be present. Less often, the patient may notice things like an unsteady gait, a deterioration of handwriting, tremor, or a certain clumsiness and impaired coordination. Occasionally, speech may be slurred and true motor weakness of the extremities will occur, but this is unusual. Symptoms like impaired concentration, slowing, apathy, and loss of interest may respond dramatically well to antidepressant medications or stimulants with significant restoration of function and the feeling of well-being. The diagnostic point of encephalopathy, however, is that this diagnosis is made when significant interference occurs with a person's occupation or activities, or, in a child, developmental milestones are delayed or not reached – such as crawling, walking, talking, etc. The later manifestations of the HIV encephalopathy show global dementia. Thus, cognitive deterioration occurs on all fronts. There is paucity of speech, sometimes to the point of mutism. Language function is impaired, with the person unable to name things or, at times, unable to speak and understand their native language. Forgetting is prominent and hallucinations may be frequent, especially visual hallucinations. Profound apathy or disinhibition may be found, similar to that found in patients with frontal lobe damage. In addition, weakness, spasticity, incoordination, and unsteadiness are common. Incontinence is also common and patients may show the signs of Parkinson's disease. The illness is also accompanied by seizures. Thus, the final state shows a patient as severely demented as any Alzheimer's patient one is likely to find in a nursing home.

In addition to the dementing process caused by the virus itself, the brain is also attacked by multiple other infections to which a person is vulnerable because immune function is impaired. These include certain primary tumors like lymphoma, which occur in the brain, or tumors which are metastatic to the brain. Occasionally, even Kaposi's sarcoma has been known to metastasize to the brain of an AIDS patient. Infections in the AIDS patients are multiple and include, in the brain, abscess, meningitis, and encephalitis. The infectious agents producing these difficulties include toxoplasma, CMV, Cryptococcus, Treponema pallidum (syphilis), multifocal leukoencephalopathy, both forms of Mycobacterium, and fungal infections.

IV. PREVENTION OF AIDS AND AIDS SPREAD

Since HIV-1 is carried in blood, plasma, body organs, sperm, and any bodily tissue, like a biopsy specimen, contact with any of these is likely to produce infection. Therefore, donated blood and plasma must be screened, and organs for transplantation must undergo the same critical inspection. Sperm banks for artificial insemination pose a significant risk for recipients unless similar donor screening is available. One infects another person by sexual intercourse, sharing of needles, and oral-genital contact. The virus is present in saliva. It is not known whether intimate kissing can spread the virus. The efficacy of condoms in preventing

TABLE 2

Universal Precautions to Prevent Transmission of HIV

Universal Precautions

Because a medical history and physical examination cannot reliably identify all patients infected with HIV or other blood-borne pathogens, blood and body-fluid precautions should be consistently used for all patients, especially those in emergency-care settings in which the risk of blood exposure is increased and the infection status of the patient is usually not known.

1. Use appropriate barrier precautions to prevent skin and mucous membrane exposure when exposure to blood, body fluids containing blood, or other body fluids to which universal precautions apply (see below) is anticipated. Wear gloves when touching blood or body fluids, mucous membranes, or nonintact skin of all patients; when handling items or surfaces soiled with blood or body fluids; and when performing venipuncture and other vascular access procedures. Change gloves after contact with each patient; do not wash or disinfect gloves for reuse. Wear masks and protective eye wear or face shields during procedures that are likely to generate droplets of blood or other body fluids to prevent exposure of mucous membranes of the mouth, nose, and eyes. Wear gowns or aprons during procedures that are likely to generate splashes of blood or other body fluids.

2. Wash hands and other skin surfaces immediately and thoroughly following contaminations with blood, body fluids containing blood, or other body fluids to which universal precautions apply. Wash hands immediately after gloves are removed.

3. Take care to prevent injuries when using needles, scalpels, and other sharp instruments or devices; when handling sharp instruments after procedures; when cleaning used instruments; and when disposing of used needles. Do not recap used needles by hand; do not remove used needles from disposable syringes by hand; and do not bend, break, or otherwise manipulate used needles by hand. Place used disposable syringes and needles, scalpel blades, and other sharp items in puncture-resistant disposal containers, which should be located as close to the use area as is practical.

4. Although saliva has not been implicated in HIV transmission, the need for emergency mouth-to-mouth resuscitation should be minimized by making mouthpieces, resuscitation bags, or other ventilation devices available for use in areas in which the need for resuscitation is predictable.

5. Health-care workers with exudative lesions or weeping dermatitis should refrain from all direct patient care and from handling patient-care equipment until the condition resolves.

Universal precautions are intended to supplement rather than replace recommendations for routine infection control, such as hand washing and use of gloves to prevent gross microbial contamination of hands. In addition, implementation of universal precautions does not eliminate the need for other category- or disease-specific isolation precautions, such as enteric precautions for infectious diarrhea or isolation for pulmonary tuberculosis. Universal precautions are not intended to change waste management programs undertaken in accordance with state and local regulations.

Body Fluids to Which Universal Precautions Apply

Universal precautions apply to blood and other body fluids containing visible blood. Blood is the single most important source of HIV, hepatitis B virus, and other blood-borne pathogens in the occupational setting. Universal precautions also apply to tissues, semen, vaginal secretions, and the following fluids: cerebrospinal, synovial, pleural, peritoneal, pericardial, and amniotic.

Universal precautions do not apply to feces, nasal secretions, sputum, sweat, tears, urine, and vomitus unless they contain visible blood. Universal precautions also do not apply to human breast milk, although gloves may be worn by health-care workers in situations in which exposure to breast milk might be frequent. In addition, universal precautions do not apply to saliva. Gloves need not be worn when feeding patients or wiping saliva from skin, although special precau-

tions are recommended for dentistry, in which contamination of saliva with blood is predictable. The risk of transmission of HIV, as well as hepatitis B virus, from these fluids and materials is extremely low or nonexistent.

Use of Gloves for Phlebotomy

Gloves should be effective in reducing the incidence of blood contamination of hands during phlebotomy (drawing of blood samples), but they cannot prevent penetrating injuries caused by needles or other sharp instruments. In universal precautions, all blood is assumed to be potentially infectious for blood-borne pathogens. Some institutions have relaxed recommendations for the use of gloves for phlebotomy by skilled health-care workers in settings in which the prevalence of blood-borne pathogens is known to be very low (e.g., volunteer blood-donation centers). Institutions that judge that routine use of gloves for all phlebotomies is not necessary should periodically reevaluate their policy. Gloves should always be available for those who wish to use them for phlebotomy. In addition, the following general guidelines apply:

1. Use gloves for performing phlebotomy if cuts, scratches, or other breaks in the skin are present.

2. Use gloves in situations in which contamination with blood may occur—for example, when performing phlebotomy on an uncooperative patient.

3. Use gloves for performing finger or heel sticks on infants and children.

4. Use gloves when training persons to do phlebotomies.

Precautions for Laboratories

Blood and other body fluids from all patients should be considered infective. To supplement the universal precautions listed above, the following precautions are recommended for workers in clinical laboratories:

1. Put all specimens of blood and body fluids in a well-constructed container with a secure lid to prevent leakage during transport. Take care when collecting each specimen to avoid contaminating the outside of the container or the laboratory form accompanying the specimen.

2. Wear gloves when processing blood and body-fluid specimens (e.g., when removing tops from vacuum tubes). Wear masks and protective eye wear if it is anticipated that mucous membranes will come in contact with blood or body fluids. Change gloves and wash hands after completion of specimen processing.

3. For routine procedures, such as histologic and pathologic studies or microbiologic culturing, a biologic safety cabinet is not necessary. However, use a biologic safety cabinet (class I or II) when procedures are conducted that have a high potential for generating droplets, such as blending, sonicating, and vigorous mixing.

4. Use a mechanical pipetting device for manipulating all liquids in the laboratory. Do not pipette by mouth.

5. Limit use of needles and syringes to situations in which there is no alternative.

6. Decontaminate work surfaces with an appropriate chemical germicide after a spill of blood or other body fluids and after work is completed.

7. Decontaminate materials contaminated during laboratory tests before reprocessing them. Place contaminated materials for disposal in bags and discard in accordance with institutional policies for disposal of infective waste.

8. Decontaminate and clean scientific equipment that has been contaminated by blood or body fluids if repair in the laboratory or transport to the manufacturer is necessary.

9. Wash hands after completing laboratory work and remove protective clothing before leaving the laboratory.

Implementation of universal precautions eliminates the need for warning labels on specimens because blood and body fluids from all patients should be considered infective.

Rubin RH. Op. cit. (p. 13).

TABLE 3

Recommendations for Screening Donated Blood and Plasma for Antibody to HIV

Initial Testing

Persons accepted as donors should be informed that their blood or plasma will be tested for HIV antibody Persons not wishing to have their blood or plasma tested must refrain from donation. Donors should be told that they will be notified if their test is positive and that they may be placed on the collection facility's donor deferral list. as is currently practiced with other infectious diseases. and should be informed of the identities of additional deferral lists to which the positive donors may be added.

All blood plasma should be tested for HIV antibody by ELISA. Any blood or plasma that is positive on initial testing must not be transfused or manufactured into other products capable of transmitting infectious agents.

When the ELISA test is used to screen populations in whom the prevalence of HIV infections is low, the proportion of positive results that are falsely positive will be high. Therefore. the ELISA test should be repeated on all seropositive specimens before the donor is notified. If the repeat ELISA test is negative, the specimen should be tested by another technique.

Other Testing

Other tests have included immunofluorescence and radio-immunoprecipitation assays, but the most extensive experience has been with the Western blot technique, in which antibodies to HIV proteins of specific molecular weights can be detected. Based on available data, the Western blot should be considered positive for antibody to HIV if band p24 or gp41 is present (alone or in combination with other bands).

Notification of Donors

If the repeat ELISA test is positive or if other tests are positive. it is the responsibility of the collection facility to ensure that the donor is notified. The information should be given to the donor by an individual especially aware of the sensitivities involved. At present, the proportion of these seropositive donors who have been infected with HIV is not known. It is. therefore. important to emphasize to the donor that the positive result is a preliminary finding that may not represent true infection. To determine the significance of a positive test, the donor should be referred to a physician for evaluation. The information should be given to the donor in a manner to ensure confidentiality of the results and of the donor's identity.

Maintaining Confidentiality

Physicians. laboratory and nursing personnel. and others should recognize the importance of maintaining confidentiality of positive test results. Disclosure of this information for purposes other than medical or public health concerns could lead to serious consequences for the individual. Screening procedures should be designed with safeguards to protect against unauthorized disclosure. Donors should be given a clear explanation of how information about them will be handled. Facilities should consider developing contingency plans in the event that disclosure is sought through legal processes. If donor deferral lists are kept, it is necessary to maintain confidentiality of such lists. Whenever appropriate, as an additional safeguard, donor deferral lists should be general, without indication of the reason for inclusion.

Medical Evaluation

The evaluation might include ELISA testing of a follow-up serum specimen and Western blot testing, if the specimen is positive Persons who continue to show serologic evidence of HIV infection should be questioned about possible exposure to the virus or possible risk factors for AIDS in the individual or his or her sexual contacts and examined for signs of AIDS or related conditions. such as lymphadenopathy, oral candidiasis. Kaposi's sarcoma. and unexplained weight loss. Additional laboratory studies might include tests for other sexually transmitted diseases. tests of immune function. and where available. tests for the presence of the virus, such as viral culture. Testing for antibodies to HIV in the individual's sexual contacts may also be useful in establishing whether the test results truly represent infection.

Recommendations for the Individual

An individual judged most likely to have an HIV infection should be provided the following information and advice:

1. The long-term prognosis for an individual infected with HIV is not known. However. data available from studies conducted among homosexual men indicate that most persons will remain infected.

2. Although asymptomatic. these individuals may transmit HIV to others. Regular medical evaluation and follow-up are advised. especially for individuals who acquire signs or symptoms suggestive of AIDS.

3. Refrain from donating blood, plasma, body organs, other tissue, or sperm.

4. There is a risk of infecting others by sexual intercourse. sharing of needles. and possibly, exposure of others to saliva through oral-genital contact or intimate kissing. The efficacy of condoms in preventing infection with HIV is unproved. but the consistent use of them may reduce transmission.

5. Toothbrushes, razors. or other implements that could become contaminated with blood should not be shared.

6. Women with a seropositive test. or women whose sexual partner is seropositive. are themselves at increased risk of acquiring AIDS If they become pregnant, their offspring are also at increased risk of acquiring AIDS.

7. After accidents resulting in bleeding, contaminated surfaces should be cleaned with household bleach freshly diluted 1:10 in water.

8. Devices that have punctured the skin, such as hypodermic and acupuncture needles. should be steam sterilized by autoclave before reuse or safely discarded. Whenever possible, disposable needles and equipment should be used.

9. When seeking medical or dental care for intercurrent illness, these persons should inform those responsible for their care of their positive antibody status so that appropriate evaluation can be undertaken and precautions taken to prevent transmission to others.

10. Testing for HIV antibody should be offered to persons who may have been infected as a result of their contact with seropositive individuals (e.g., sexual partners. persons with whom needles have been shared, or infants born to seropositive mothers).

Rubin RH. Op. cit. (p. 11).

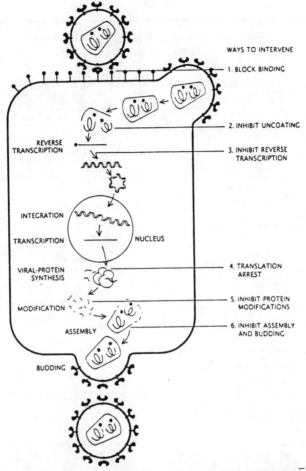

WAYS TO INTERVENE

1. BLOCK BINDING

2. INHIBIT UNCOATING

REVERSE
TRANSCRIPTION

3. INHIBIT REVERSE
TRANSCRIPTION

INTEGRATION

TRANSCRIPTION   NUCLEUS

VIRAL-PROTEIN
SYNTHESIS

4. TRANSLATION
ARREST

5. INHIBIT PROTEIN
MODIFICATIONS

MODIFICATION

6. INHIBIT ASSEMBLY
AND BUDDING

ASSEMBLY

BUDDING

HIV LIFE CYCLE is subject to attack by drugs at several stages. Certain antibodies could block the binding of the viral envelope glycoprotein, gp120, to CD4 receptors on the surface of helper *T* cells (*1*). Other agents might keep viral RNA and reverse transcriptase from escaping their protein coat (*2*). Drugs such as AZT and other dideoxynucleosides prevent the reverse transcription of viral RNA into viral DNA (*3*). Later on, antisense oligonucleotides could block the translation of mRNA into viral proteins (*4*). Before they can be assembled, viral proteins must be modified: certain compounds could interfere with such processes as the cleavage of proteins or the addition of sugar groups (*5*). Finally, such antiviral substances as interferons could keep the virus particle from assembling itself and budding out of the cell (*6*).

Fig. 5. Yarchoan R, Mitsuya H, Broder S. AIDS therapies. In *Scientific American* (vol. 259, no. 4), 110–119 (p. 112).

infection is unproved. Receptive anal intercourse is generally thought to be one of the most dangerous forms of sexual contact. Toothbrushes, razors, or other implements that could become contaminated with blood should not be shared. Whenever possible, disposable needles and equipment should be used. If equipment is to be used again, such as hypodermic and acupuncture needles, these should be autoclaved before they are reused. Whenever accidents result in bleeding, contaminated surfaces should be cleaned with household bleach freshly diluted 1: 10 in water.

Tables 2 and 3 present the recommendations for screening donated blood and plasma for antibody to HIV and universal precautions to prevent transmission of HIV.

PRESENT AND FUTURE TREATMENTS FOR AIDS

Figure 5 shows several intervention points in the life of the viral particle. Depicted are the points at which an intervention could be designed. Currently, AZT is the most effective treatment for AIDS. It was synthesized by Jerome Horowitz in 1964 at the Michigan Cancer Foundation.

It is important to know that the use of AZT has basically changed the clinical picture of AIDS. Thanks to this new agent, the manifestations of the disease are less severe and the patient is generally able to maintain a healthy status longer than was possible before. Even in the patient with a dementing syndrome caused by the virus, AZT has been shown to restore brain function to a higher level. Yarchoan et al. discovered in February of 1985 that this agent, synthesized more than 20 years earlier, could inhibit HIV replication. Only five months later the drug was administered to the first patient in the clinical center at the National Institutes of Health. AZT inhibits reverse transcriptase, causing the viral replicating machine to insert a "dud" in the nucleotide sequence, making further replication, and therefore infection, impossible. At the present time it appears that AZT increases the median survival time of patients with advanced AIDS by about one year. It was, in fact, this evidence that caused the Food and Drug Administration in the United States to approve AZT in March of 1987 as a prescription drug for severe HIV infection. If given early in the course of HIV infection, about the time when the level of T4 helper lymphocytes has fallen to 500, it will significantly slow the progression of AIDS in most persons, both by its direct antiviral effect and by partially restoring immune function. The helper T4 cell from patients given AZT appears to be better able to kill HIV-infected cells.

In the case of HIV encephalopathy, it is possible to demonstrate at least temporary improvement with AZT, and improvement is apparent within the first few weeks of therapy. This improvement is demonstrated by detailed neuropsychological testing. In some cases it can be shown that the IQ, which invariably falls during HIV encephalopathy, returns to normal levels during treatment.

Some of the limitations of AZT include the short period of time it stays in the blood. Very large oral doses must be given every six hours in order to maintain a plasma concentration which is therapeutic, i.e., above one micromole/liter. Moreover, AZT can have its own toxic effect on the marrow, such that patients become gradually anemic and at times require a blood transfusion. In other cases, especially at higher doses, white blood cell production is impaired and, with that, immune competence is further damaged.

The use of prophylactic aerosolized pentamidine can also delay the appearance of AIDS in an infected individual.

Some new treatments, such as deoxyinosine (DDI; Videx) and deoxycytidine (DDC) act in exactly the same fashion as AZT, causing reverse transcriptase to incorporate a bogus nucleotide, thereby becoming incompetent. These two drugs are already in experimental use in the United States, appear to be less toxic than AZT, and may be valuable either as a substitute for AZT or in combination with it. Another treatment, recombinant soluble CD4, binds the gp120 protein, essentially fooling it into believing that it is hooked onto a T cell. This drug also has been used in AIDS patients, is well tolerated, and is also helpful at least in slowing the progression and severity of the infection.

Finally, a group of physicians recently reported that extracorporeal photopheresis, a method in which patients take a photosensitizing drug called 8-methoxypsoralen, then have their lymphocytes isolated, exposed to ultraviolet A light and returned to them, produced rather dramatic benefit in 4 of 5 patients with AIDS-related complex. (Bisaccia *et al.*, AIM, 1990: 270–75) Blood cultures for HIV became negative in 3 patients, though in one became again positive at 15 months.

Because of the ethical interests of the FICU International Group for the Study of Bioethics, a summary policy statement on AIDS is included (Table 4), covering important issues such as the obligation of physicians and other health care professionals and hospitals to provide competent

TABLE 4

Summary Policy Statement on AIDS

1. The American College of Physicians and the Infectious Diseases Society of America believe that physicians, other health-care professionals, and hospitals are obligated to provide competent and humane care to all patients, including patients with AIDS and AIDS-related conditions as well as HIV-infected patients with unrelated medical problems. The denial of appropriate care to patients for any reason is unethical.

2. Physicians and other health-care professionals are urged to become fully aware of potential risks and problems encountered in caring for HIV-positive patients and patients with AIDS and to take appropriate steps to minimize them. Such problems include the risks of HIV transmission, economic problems, and personal psychologic stresses.

3. Elected leaders, employers, community service organizations, welfare agencies, public housing authorities, prison officials, and school officials are urged to become fully informed and educate others about HIV infection and, particularly, to understand the limited mechanisms by which the virus can be transmitted. Dissemination of such knowledge should serve to guide public policy development, to alleviate discrimination against those who become infected with the virus, and to limit the further spread of infection.

4. Testing for HIV antibody should be used only when it will benefit the patient or contacts to whom the virus may have been transmitted or for protection of the public health.

5. Counseling and educational efforts, rather than policies promoting physical restriction or quarantine, are appropriate methods for controlling the spread of HIV infection.

6. The confidentiality of patients infected with HIV should be protected to the greatest extent possible, consistent with the duty to protect others and to protect the public health.

7. Physicians should incorporate into their practices standard procedures for taking complete sexual histories of their patients and should assume responsibility for candid communication with and education of persons known to be at risk for HIV infection. The need to modify sexual practices to prevent transmission of infection should be stressed. In addition, physicians are urged to take a major part in educating the public to eliminate misconceptions about AIDS.

8. The American College of Physicians and the Infectious Diseases Society of America encourage continued research into the causes, prevention, and treatment of AIDS and AIDS-related conditions. In addition to biomedical aspects, research into psychosocial and economic issues related to AIDS should be increased. Studies of the effectiveness of various types of educational interventions on behavior modification are critically important.

Rubin RH. Op. cit. (p. 15).

and humane care to all AIDS patients. Duties of physicians and health care professionals to educate both the public and AIDS patients are also outlined. Statements are made about testing for HIV, counseling and education rather than quarantine for control of AIDS, patient confidentiality, physician responsibility, and the obligation for a continuing research into the causes, prevention and treatment of AIDS and AIDS-related condition.

NOTES

Tables 1, 2, 3, and 4, in *The HIV Infection*, are from R. H. Rubin, "Acquired immunodeficiency syndrome", in *Scientific American Medicine*, E. Rubenstein (ed.), 1989, *Annals of Internal Medicine*.

Figure 1, in *The HIV Infection* is an illustration in "AIDS 1988", by R.C. Gallo and L. Montagnier, in *Scientific American*, October 1988, p. 43.

Figure 2, *in The HIV Infection*, is an illustration in "The Moleclar Biology of the AIDS Virus" by W. A. Haseltine and F. Wong-Staal, in *Scientific American*, October 1988, p. 51.

Figure 3, in *The HIV Infection*, is an illustration, by Ian Worpole, in "HIV Infection: The Clinical Picture," by R. Redfield and D. Burke, in *Scientific American*, October 1988, p. 97.

Figure 4, in *The HIV Infection*, is an illustration by Ian Worpole, in "HIV Infection: The Clinical Picture," by R. Redfield and D. Burke, in *Scientific American*, October 1988, p. 94.

Figure 5, in *The HIV Infection*, is an illustration, by Hank Iken, in "AIDS Therapies", by R. Yarchoan, H. Mitsuya, and S. Broder, in *Scientific American*, October 1988, p. 112.

BIBLIOGRAPHY

Bisaccia, E., Berger C. and Klainer, A. S.: 1990, 'Extracorporeal photopheresis in the treatment of AIDS-related complex: A pilot study', *Annals of Internal Medicine* 113, 270–275.

Chu, S. Y., Buehler, J. W. and Berkelman, R. L.: 1990, 'Impact of the humanimmunodeficiency virus epidemic on mortality in women of reproductive age, United States' *The Journal of American Medical Association* 264, 225–229.

Dalakas, M., Wichman, A. and Sever, J.: 1989, 'AIDS and the nervous system',*The Journal of American Medical Association* 261, 2396–2399.

Fahey, J. L., Taylor, J. M. G., Detels, R. *et al.*: 1990, 'The prognostic value ofcellular and serologic markers in infection with human immunodeficiency virus type 1', *The New England Journal of Medicine* 322, 166–172.

Ho, D. D., Bredesen, D. E., Vinters, H. V. *et al.*: 1989, 'The acquired immunodeficiency syndrome (AIDS) dementia complex', *Annals of Internal Medicine* 111, 400–410.

Navia, B. A. and Price, R. W.: 1987, 'The acquired immunodeficiency syndrome dementia complex as the presenting or sole manifestation of human immunodeficiency virus infection', *Archives of Neurology* 44, 65–69.

Osmond, D.: International epidemiology of AIDS. AIDS KnowledgeBase from San Francisco General Hospital. Updated September 1990.

Pizzo, P. A.: 1989, 'Emerging concepts in the treatment of HIV infection in children', *The Journal of the American Medical Association* 262, 1989–1992.

Rubin, R. H.: 1989, Acquired immunodeficiency syndrome. In: Rubenstein, E., Federman, D. D. (eds.), *Scientific American Medicine* 7.XI.1–20, New York: Scientific American

Scientific American, AIDS, volume 259, number 4, 1988, entire issue.

PORTER STOREY

ARTIFICIAL FEEDING AND HYDRATION
IN ADVANCED ILLNESS

In most people's final weeks of prolonged illness, their appetite and strength decline. In this culture, where we often show our affection and concern for each other with food, it is very distressing to see a loved one not eat. Many articles have been written on the question of whether it is ethical to withhold artificially administered food and fluids from dying patients. An important basis for making such decisions is the understanding of what such treatment entails (the "costs") and how much good they do (the "benefits"). This is the subject of this essay.

"Advanced illness", for the discussion that follows, will be defined as the final weeks of an incurable illness like cancer or the progressive failure of a vital organ like the heart, lungs, kidney, liver, or brain. It is usually characterized by progressive debilitation – the patient spends nearly all of his time in bed. There are certainly very serious conditions, such as automobile accidents, burns, or following abdominal surgery, when artificially supplied food and fluids are unquestionably of benefit. In these situations, unlike advanced illnesses, a period of intensive treatment can completely restore the health of the patient.

What is involved in artificially (i.e., through a tube) supplying a patient with food and water? What are the "costs" of this treatment to the patient? There are four common ways of accomplishing artificial feeding. The most common method is to push a tube the size of a pencil through the nose, down the throat, and into the stomach – a nasogastric tube. To accomplish this, the hands of a confused or "uncooperative" patient are tied to the bedrails. The head is held tightly by one person and a second person pushes the plastic tube, dripping with lubricant, into the nose. When the tube hits the back of the nasal passage, the nasopharynx, it is quite painful. To get the tube to turn downward it must be pushed hard against this sensitive part of the upper throat. As the tube turns (hopefully) downwards, it pushes against the back of the throat and frequently the patient gags and vomits. Sometimes the tube emerges from the mouth or nose and the procedure must begin again. If the patient is alert and very cooperative he or she can attempt to drink water while the

67

K.Wm. Wildes (ed.), Birth, Suffering and Death, 67–75.
© 1992 *Kluwer Academic Publishers. Printed in the Netherlands.*

tube is being pushed down the throat. This helps direct the tube into the stomach. If the patient cannot do this the tube often ends up in the lungs and the procedure begins again. Hopefully the tube ends up in the stomach and the position is determined by applying suction and obtaining gastric juice from the stomach. Air is pushed through the tube and the nurse listens for a gurgling sound over the stomach. If the nurse guesses wrong about the correct placement of the tube, or later if the patient coughs or vomits up the end of the tube, the feedings will go into the lungs instead of the stomach – which causes "aspiration pneumonia", a serious lung infection which is often fatal.

If the patient is very cooperative and the nurse is very skillful, a small (1/8 inch) diameter, soft flexible tube can be inserted which is not uncomfortable once it is placed. Unfortunately most of the patients who get nasogastric tubes in their final weeks are not so cooperative, and the small soft tubes are harder to place, harder to use for suction (emptying the stomach), and easily plugged by the thick feedings. Many patients, therefore get the larger, stiff tubes that are more painful to have pushed down, and quite uncomfortable to have in. The tubes must be secured to the nose or forehead with tape (which is irritating and very undignified). Since the tubes irritate the nose and throat, many patients reach up and (consciously or unconsciously) pull them out. The entire painful insertion procedure must then begins again. After a patient pulls the tube out a few times, his or her hands are left tied to the bedrails so he cannot turn over or get comfortable in bed. Many patients develop bedsores because they are tied in one position in bed and cannot even get to the toilet. The present acute shortage of nurses insures that a patient, thus restrained, will spend a substantial part of his day sitting in his own urine and stool. The patient can still move his nose down to his tied hand and frequently pulls out the nasogastric tube despite such restraints.

Because of the many problems and discomforts of nasogastric tubes, methods of putting tubes directly through the skin of the upper abdomen and into the stomach were developed. Initially the gastrostomy tubes were inserted under general anesthesia, but many patients are too sick to tolerate being put to sleep. The most common method today for inserting tubes directly into the stomach is with the patient awake but sleepy from medication, like Valium, and a mild pain reliever. The patient must swallow a large tube, about 3/4 inch in diameter, called a gastroscope. The doctor can look through this scope to make sure the end of the scope has reached the stomach. The scope has a light on the end of it and when it is pushed out against the abdominal wall, the doctor "stabs" the patient's abdomen where he sees the light. The gastrostomy tube is then inserted right through that stab wound. The wound causes pain for several days. Although expensive and uncomfortable to insert, the gastrostomy tube is considered more humane for long term artificial feedings.

Nasogastric and gastrostomy tubes are preferred for artificial feedings because large quantities of protein, fats, and sugars can be infused through them. The feeding formulas need not be sterile so they are less expensive and the apparatus can often be managed at home or in a nursing home. The large quantities of rich feedings often over-stretch the stomach so that cramping pain and vomiting are common. Many ill patients do not absorb the concentrated feedings and frequently episodes of diarrhea make this uncomfortable procedure even more intolerable for a bedbound patient.

Is this method of feeding safe? In a study of seventy patients in a skilled nursing facility physically connected to a tertiary care hospital (i.e., ideal conditions), Dr. Ciocon et al. noted the following rate of complications (Ciocon et al., 1988):

	Nasogastric		Gastrostomy	
	<2wks	2wk–11mo.	<2wks	2wk–11mo.
Self Extubation	67%	39%	44%	0
Aspiration Pneumonia	43%	44%	56%	56%
Misplacement	2%	0	6%	6%
Leak at Insertion Site	0	0	13%	13%
Infected at Insertion Site	0	0	19%	13%
Peritonitis	0	0	6%	0
Clogged Tube	2%	20%	50%	38%
Kinked Tube	4%	6%	0	0
Difficulty in Insertion	7%	4%	6%	19%
At least one of the above	70%	65%	94%	88%

The third method frequently employed to artificially administer fluid and nutrients is the peripheral intravenous line. This method requires that a needle or tiny plastic tube be stuck through the skin into the vein, usually on the forearm or hand. This method is clearly the least invasive but it is not without risks and discomforts. The needle must be re-inserted every day or two because it becomes dislodged, infected or inflamed in a short time. The hand must frequently be immobilized and the patient's movement is restricted by the necessity of always staying near the IV pole. Blood clots, local infections, and infiltrations of fluid outside the vein are common painful complications. As veins get harder to find, the stabbing with needles becomes more frequent and uncomfortable as sites on the legs or the neck are employed. Despite these problems this method remains the most common for fluid administration. Only vitamins and low concentrations of fats and sugars can be given by this route because higher concentrations of nutrients and amino acids are too irritating to peripheral veins.

To overcome this limitation, central venous lines were developed. These plastic tubes are inserted under the collar bone or into the base of the neck and extend down to the heart. These tubes are more dangerous than any of the above methods because it is so easy to puncture and collapse a lung when inserting the tube and because the infections and blood clots they often cause are life-threatening. They are routinely used in surgery and intensive care units and can be left in place much longer than peripheral IV lines. They are more uncomfortable to have inserted than peripheral IV lines because the tubes (and thus the hole in the skin through which they are passed) are larger. Once inserted they are not uncomfortable. Concentrated solutions of amino acids, sugars, fats, and vitamins can then be put directly into the bloodstream. Infections around the central venous catheters or from contamination of the sterile fluids are common and require re-hospitalization for IV antibiotics. The cost of just four months of this "hyperalimentation" (or total parenteral nutrition) would pay for an entire college education at a fine private institution (see Bole, this volume).

There are social and psychological costs of these treatments as well. Meal times are social gatherings and enjoyable for most people. Since appetite is completely suppressed by the artificial feeding, and the patient is tied to a bag of fluid and a delivery pump, he misses out on these most important times. Sometimes the only human contact a nursing home patient gets is being fed. With a tube and a pump, even this is taken away.

The most serious "costs" of artificial feeding and hydration are related to the effects of the nutrients and fluids themselves. As vital organs become diseased, they are less able to accommodate stresses like those imposed by artificial feeding. For example, a patient with congestive heart failure may be quite comfortable on the little he feels like eating or drinking. If he is given a large volume of tube feeding or IV fluid, his ailing heart decompensates. The fluid collects in his ankles and legs causing uncomfortable edema and may even collect in his lungs. Too much fluid in the lungs is called pulmonary edema and is extremely distressing and life-threatening for the patient. Likewise when the kidneys fail, the fluids cannot be excreted and these same symptoms occur from fluid overload. The protein in artificial feeding rapidly increases the blood urea nitrogen and makes the renal failure patient nauseated and confused. A failing liver usually causes fluid to collect in the abdomen. This excess fluid, called ascites, is very uncomfortable to carry around and can even restrict a patient's ability to breath. Artificial feeding or IV fluids accelerates the development of ascites. The protein load from artificial feedings can increase the blood ammonia levels in hepatic (liver) failure which causes confusion, delirium, and finally stupor and coma. Failing lungs are often not able to get rid of the mucous they make. Frequent coughing and shortness of breath results from the increased mucous and lung water which is produced when a patient with emphysema or pneumonia gets artificial feedings.

Cancer patients nearly all lose their appetites and lose weight. In 1955 Drs. Terepka and Waterhouse at the University of Rochester evaluated eight cancer patients before and after force-feeding them on a special metabolism ward. They found that in half the patients the forced feedings accelerated the growth of the cancer irreversibly (Terepka and Waterhouse, 1956). In mammary tumors implanted into rats (Buzby *et al.*, 1980) or petri dishes (Stragand *et al.*, 1979), in rats inoculated with carcinosarcoma (Daly *et al.*, 1980; Reynolds *et al.*, 1980) or hepatoma (Cameron, 1981; Popp *et al.*, 1981), or rats who developed a sarcoma from methylcholanthrene exposure (Lowry *et al.*, 1979), *tumor growth was* slowed by restricted diets and *accelerated by artificial feeding* (total parenteral nutrition). Sensitive biochemical measurements indicate that cancers in humans are also accelerated by intravenous feedings (Ota *et al.*, 1986). When the data was pooled from twenty-eight controlled trials of total parenteral nutrition (TPN) in cancer patients, Klein *et al.* found that TPN caused an increased incidence of infections and a decreased response from chemotherapy (Klein *et al.*, 1986). The American College of Physicians carefully reviewed this subject and concluded that artificial feedings make cancer patients die faster "... parenteral nutritional support was associated with net harm, and no conditions could be defined in which such treatment appeared to be of benefit" (ACP, 1989).

The patient's family must also carry a heavier burden when artificial feedings are used during the final weeks. It's hard enough to be anticipating the loss of a loved one. Medicare and insurance regulations now require most patients to spend their last weeks at home, so the family will become the caregiver. They must learn how to regulate, clean, and operate the tubes and pumps. They must pay the exorbitant cost of the solutions and equipment, which may cut deeply into money set aside for a college education or retirement. The increased fluid intake will mean more incontinence, vomiting, and diarrhea in a bedbound patient – a heavy burden for an elderly spouse or a daughter, who must also care for her own family. The pumps are usually run through the night so these distressing problems often happen in the middle of the night. Worst of all is the guilt they feel. The patient has no appetite and usually hates the tubes and feedings but the doctor has made it the family's responsibility. When the patient continues to get weaker and lose weight, whose fault is it? No wonder so many people end up in nursing homes!

Are there not benefits of artificial feedings that outweigh these high costs for dying patients? Don't these feedings help them live longer? As discussed above, tube feedings often accelerate the disease process or cause fatal complications like sepsis (bacteria in the bloodstream) or aspiration pneumonia (feeding solution poured into the lungs). In a survey of elderly patients in a New York community-based teaching hospital, Dr. Quill found that 64 % of patients treated with nasogastric tubes died in the hospital and 53 % had to be tied down to keep the tubes in (Quill, 1989).

Isn't it important to prevent dehydration and electrolyte (sodium, potassium, calcium, etc.) imbalance when people stop eating? This is often the excuse given for treating dying patients with IV fluids. At St. Christopher's Hospice in London, where artificial feedings and hydration are not used, twenty-two patients with advanced cancer died within 48 hours (12 within 24 hours) of having a blood test. Twelve had essentially normal electrolytes and the other ten had elevated urea or calcium levels. All died peacefully, without distress (Oliver, 1984). Thus fears of some calamity from dehydration or electrolyte imbalance should not force dying patients to have unwanted tubes and needles.

Is it not necessary to use artificial feedings and fluids for comfort? As discussed above, having a tube pushed down one's throat and one's hands tied down to keep it in is anything but comfortable. A Seattle hospice nurse has described how often IV fluids lead to the use of urinary catheters for incontinence, suction tubes pushed down the trachea to remove excess mucous, nasogastric suction tubes to control vomiting, and needles put in the abdomen to drain ascites (Zerwekh, 1983). When ninety-six hospice nurses in New Jersey and Pennsylvania were recently surveyed, 82 % said that dehydration was not painful, and 73 % said dehydrated dying patients rarely complain of thirst, while only 1 % thought that dry mouth from lack of fluids necessitate the use of IVs and/or tube feedings (Andrews and Levine, 1989). They know how easily this one common symptom of dehydration is palliated by small sips of water from a syringe, ice chips or a room humidifier. No wonder prominent physicians dedicated to comforting the dying, in both Britain (Baines, 1978; Lamerton, 1980) and the United States (Printz, 1988; Billings, 1985), have opposed the use of artificially administered food and fluids.

But is it not "unnatural" to stop feeding someone? Loss of appetite and weight loss are part of our body's defense against disease. Cachectin (also called tumor necrosis factor because it fights cancer) is a hormone that our immune system produces when we are attacked by a variety of tumors and infections (Tracey *et al.*, 1989). In addition to curbing the appetite, and thus preventing the above mentioned problems, it helps remodel damaged tissue and stimulates the body's fight against infections and tumors (Goh, 1990).

Why are artificial feedings so often given to patients with advanced illnesses? Doctors feel guilty that they cannot cure the illness and fearful of lawsuits if they don't "do something". Hospitals fear that Medicare and insurance companies won't pay the bill unless "something was done". Families feel guilty about not being able to care for the patient at home and want their patient to get "all the best treatment," or at least "what can be done". Nursing homes refuse admission to chronically ill patients with poor appetites who don't have feeding tubes. They fear lawsuits or regulatory agency penalty for "starving the patient to death".

This is one area of science that doesn't need more clinical trials. Some years ago this author spent many hours designing a randomized trial of IV fluids for comfort in terminally ill patients. My institution's review board felt it would be unethical to submit dying patients to uncomfortable, problematic, even dangerous treatments (IV fluids) with no expected benefit. The appropriate treatment for guilt is education. We must teach our doctors, hospitals, families, and nursing homes that "doing something" isn't always right and can be very wrong. The appropriate treatment for fear is courage. We must stand up against this barbaric custom and allow our patients to die with the comfort and dignity they deserve.

BIBLIOGRAPHY

American College of Physicians: 1989, 'Parenteral nutrition in patients receiving cancer chemotherapy', *Annals of Internal Medicine*, 110, 734–736.

Andrews, M. R. and Levine, A. M.: 1989, 'Dehydration in the terminal patient: Perception of hospice nurses', *American Journal of Hospice Care*, 31–34.36.

Baines, M. J.: 1978, 'Control of other symptoms', in Saunders, C. M. (ed.), *The Management of Terminal Disease*, Chicago, Year Book Medical Publishers.

Billings, J. A.: 1985, 'Comfort measures for the terminally ill – Is dehydration painful?', *Journal of The American Gerontology Society*, 33, 808–810.

Buzby, G. P., Mullen, J. L. and Stein, T. P.: 1980, 'Host-tumor interaction and nutrient supply', *Cancer*, 45, 2940–2948.

Cameron, I. L.: 1981, 'Effect of total parenteral nutrition on tumor-host response in rats', *Cancer Treatment Report* (Suppl 5), 93–99.

Ciocon, J. O., Silverstone, F. A., Graver. M. *et al.*: 1988, 'Tube feeding in elderly patients, indications, benefits, and complications', *Archives of Internal Medicine* 148, 429–433.

Daly, J. M., Copeland, E. M., Dudrick, S. J. *et al.*: 1980, 'Nutritional repletion of malnourished tumor-bearing and nontumor-bearing rats', *Journal of Surgical Research*, 28, 507–518.

Goh, C. R.: 1990, 'Tumor necrosis factors in clinical practice', *Annual of the Academy of Medicine – Singapore*, 19, 235–239.

Klein, S., Simes. J. and Blackburn, G. L.: 1986, 'Total parenteral nutrition and cancer clinical trials', *Cancer*, 58, 1378–1386.

Lamerton, R.: 1980, *Care of the Dying*, New York, Penguin Books.

Lowry, S. F., Goodgame, J. T. Jr., Norton, J. A. *et al.*: 1979, 'Effect of chronic protein malnutrition on host-tumor composition and growth. *Journal of Surgical Research*, 26, 79–86.

Oliver, D.: 1984, 'Terminal dehydration', *The Lancet*, September 15.

Ota, D. M., Nishioka, K., Grossie, B. *et al.*: 1986, 'Erythrocyte polyamine levels during intravenous feeding of patients with colorectal carcinoma', *European Journal of Cancer Clinical Oncology*, 22, 837–842.

Popp, M. B., Morrison, S. D. and Brennan, M. F.: 1981, 'Total parenteral nutrition in a methylcholanthrene-induced rat sarcoma model', *Cancer Treatment Report* (Suppl 5), 137–143.

Printz, L. A.: 1988, 'Is withholding hydration a valid comfort measure in the terminally ill', *Geriatrics*, 43, 84–88.

Quill, T. E.: 1989, 'Utilization of nasogastric feeding tubes in a group of chronically ill, elderly patients in a community hospital' *Achieves of Internal Medicine*, 149, 1937–1941.

Reynolds, H. M., Daly, J. M., Rowlands, B. J. *et al.*: 1980, 'Effects of nutritional repletion on host and tumor response to chemotherapy', *Cancer*, 45, 3069–3074.

Stragand, J. J., Braunschweiger, P. G., Pollice, A. A. *et al.*: 1979, 'Cell kinetic alterations in murine mammary tumors following fasting and refeeding', *European Journal Cancer*, 15, 281–286.

Terepka, A. R. and Waterhouse, C.: 1956, 'Metabolic observations during the forced

feeding of patients with cancer', *American Journal of Medicine* 225–238.
Tracey, K. J., Vlassara, H. and Ceramie, A.: 1989, 'Cachectin/Tumor necrosis factor', *The Lancet*, May 20, 1122–1126.
Zerwekh, J. V.: 1983, 'The dehydration question', *Nursing*, 13(1), 47–51.

SECTION II

THEOLOGICAL PERSPECTIVES

ANTONIO AUTIERO

DIGNITY, SOLIDARITY, AND THE SANCTITY OF HUMAN LIFE

In many discussions of the human tragedies and choices which are often linked to the ethical issues of death and dying, phrases such as "the sanctity of life", "the dignity of human life", and "human solidarity" are often invoked as part of the discussion. Such phrases are used in a number of ways. At times they are deployed to prohibit actions. Those, for example, who argue for restrictions on abortion often speak of the sanctity and the dignity of human life. At the same time such language is used in appeals which are deployed to support injunctions to act in ways that are supportive of others. Such injunctions are supported by the appeal to "solidarity" among human beings. Indeed much of the social teaching of the Church, exhorting the fulfillment of positive moral obligations towards others, invokes a language of "solidarity", "dignity", and "sanctity".

While this language is widely used in many contexts it is often not clearly understood. Like many other fragments of moral language drawn from classical, Christian culture, the language of "dignity", "solidarity", and "sanctity" is open to a wide array of interpretations once the language is removed from its original context. Such contextual changes present at least two dangers for the Church. First, as confusion grows in the secular world about the meaning of such language, the faithful may themselves become confused about what this language means and what can be concluded from it. Second, if Catholics engage in discussions in the secular world about public policy issues, such as euthanasia or abortion, they will have to understand the theological roots of this language if they are to translate it creatively so that others, outside the tradition who may not share the same values, might come to understand the values it expresses. The goal of this essay is simply to contextualize these phrases so that we might understand their use in the moral issues of death and dying.

K.Wm. Wildes (ed.), Birth, Suffering and Death, 79–83.
© 1992 *Kluwer Academic Publishers. Printed in the Netherlands.*

A FAMILY OF ATTITUDES

These phrases (i.e., "sanctity of life", "human dignity", "human solidarity") which are often used in moral arguments, represent a family of views and attitudes which are not often carefully articulated (Boyle, p. 221). They are not restricted to the realm of Roman Catholic moral and social thought but are also used by philosophers and ethicists in secular discussions (Clouser; Donagan). In both the Catholic and secular world this family of expressions is employed in the context of normative discourse which seeks to regulate the development of ethics in fields such as medicine, biology, economics, and genetics. Phrases such as "human dignity", "sanctity of life" and "mutual solidarity" are invoked to support important secular notions such as "human rights" (e.g., UN Declaration on human rights). However, it is not always clear what these phrases mean. The ambiguity of meaning for this family of terms has the consequence that there will also be a wide range of conclusions drawn from these terms if they function as major premises of moral arguments. While the words may sound the same, the meanings of these terms will be related to the anthropology, moral vision, and values which people presuppose in their use. It follows that other terms, such as "human rights" can have equally ambiguous meanings.

These phrases form a family relationship whose meaning is often tied to a perspective of Christian theology. This family of expressions – sanctity of life, dignity of human life, and solidarity – as commonly used in the West, find their common lineage in Christian understandings of creation and man as the "imago Dei" (Genesis 1: 26). The Fathers of the Church were influenced by the view of the Old Testament which emphasized the creation of God as being both the beginning and the destiny of man. Since *all* life is created, what is it that distinguishes human life as "sacred"? Human life has a "unique" status in that God impresses onto man His image and resemblance and therefore makes the human being above all the other beings which are His creatures but not really a mirror of the Creator. Man is part of the creation but he is also distinguished from the rest of creation as he is to rule creation. Man's dominion is not a license to exploit creation but rather a charge to rule as God would rule. All life, since it comes from God, has a sacredness about it and demands respect for it belongs to another. It belongs to God. The special dignity and sanctity of human life comes from bearing the image of God and the responsibility to rule like God.

In the human the divine is expressed in the world. Irenaeus best captures this patristic sense when he wrote: "Gloria enim Dei vivens homo, vita autem hominis visio Dei" (*Against Heresies* 4,20,7). The glory of God is the living human and the life of the human is the vision of God. In this perspective of faith, human life is made "holy" and endowed with "dignity" because of its relationship to God. Irenaeus, in speaking of the "glory" of man, is not speaking of a secular sense of "self-improvement" for the center is not the human but the Divine expressed in the human (Donovan). In the patristic era the reference to dignity had a background and application which was largely ethical. The Christian had to assume a different style in judgment and behavior from the other citizen of the Empire. These themes of the divine image and the place of human beings in creation are themes that recur a number of times in the theological and spiritual writings of the Church (e.g., Ambrose, *De dignitate conditionis humanae*, in PL 184, 485 ss).

The theme of man's divine image has been developed in different ways in the history of Christian theology and spirituality. In the reflections in the twelfth and thirteenth centuries this theme is integrated into a wider anthropology. The scholastic thinkers sought to identify which characteristic(s) distinguished human life from all other forms of bodily, created life. The epoch of scholastic philosophy was characterized by an emphasis on the intellectual and rational dimension of God's image impressed onto man. The expression "imago in specula rationis" manifests this truth. The pivotal point here is that human dignity consists in man's ability to know himself and God. In the Roman Catholic tradition human life has often been distinguished from other forms of life by the faculties of will and intellect. These faculties, unique to man in the embodied created world, were seen as the most divine of human attributes.

One can see, within the Christian tradition, different leitmotifs for interpreting concepts such as human "dignity", "solidarity" and "sanctity". Some have interpreted the "image" of God in a holistic manner where the whole of the human being is touched by the divine impress of God. While other voices in the tradition have focused on particular faculties such as intellect and will. Such particular interpretations while worthy of attention, reduce the transparency of the divine imprint onto the human creature. It concealed, moreover, the nobility of the person as a whole reducing him to a broken system of intelligence and will, reason, heart and body. Although clearly present in the Bible this holistic anthropology was obfuscated by the dualistic tendencies of Greek philosophy which themselves penetrated into primitive Christianity. The recovery of this holistic concept should be an urgent task now. The dignity of the person does not concern only his capacity for knowledge and conscience but implies also the total good of his reality, his will, his body, his interpersonal relations and at the same time his relation to God without loosing the contact with the historical situations which are always precarious and always threatened with the risk of negative and evil. One finds, within this volume attempts to present a more holistic view of human life as essential to bioethical decision making (Ashley, Schotsmans, Bader, Wildes in this volume).

The dignity of the person is dignity of the whole being because in this being there lives and acts the presence of God expressing Himself through the impression of His image. Man is thus exalted in his nature and in his history as human subject and as such is the beneficiary of basic rights and at the same time able to accomplish the corresponding duties. The dignity which belongs to him as Image of God is not derived or added but is original and intrinsic because man receives his being from God and at the same time this being is the Image of the Perfect Being. Because of the deep unity between the plan of creation and the plan of Salvation everyone has the Image of God and thus derives from this feature the basis of his dignity which expresses itself in the right to have rights and to accept duties.

This sense of human life, lived as an icon of the divine, grounds of responsibility toward others (Schotsmans, Bader, this volume). It also reinforces the sense of the "giftedness" of human life (Ashley, this volume). Finally, it leads us to understand human life as more than mere biological existence (Wildes, this volume).

LOST IN A SECULAR CONTEXT

The language of sanctity, solidarity, and dignity, has strong and particular theological grounding within the Roman Catholic Tradition. This constellation takes its meanings from the belief that human beings are made in the image of God. Those within the tradition are able to grasp the meanings of these terms because of their faith in the divine impress.

In confronting dilemmas of medical ethics it will be difficult to transpose and interpret this constellation of terms and expressions so that they can function in a secular context which does not believe that human beings mirror the divine. A secular context will lack the necessary canonical view of human life and the "good" for human beings (Engelhardt, 1991). Just as there is no canonical sense of the "good" in secular society so too there is no canonical anthropology. Such conditions, present in the post modern culture, leaves the language of "sanctity", "dignity" and "solidarity" subject to a wide variety of interpretations such that people may use the same terms but hold very different meanings. A secular world, which eschews a faith in God, will find the language of *imago dei*, at best, difficult to understand or, perhaps, meaningless. This means that the other terms will have lost their conceptual anchor and become fragmented. In public policy debates, in the post modern world, it will be ineffective for a Christian to simply invoke terms of his faith. Rather, their meanings, will be widely varied and incoherent. The task, in addressing a secular, morally pluralistic world is to find ways which convey such values and concerns.

BIBLIOGRAPHY

Boyle, J.: 1989, 'Sanctity of life and suicide: Tensions and developments within common morality', in Baruch A. Brody (ed.), *Suicide and Euthanasia*, Kluwer Academic Publishers, *Philosophy and Medicine*, Vol. 35, pp. 221–250.

Clouser, K. Danner: 1973, 'The sanctity of life – An analysis of a concept', *Annals of Internal Medicine*, 78: 119–125.

Donovan, M. A.: 1988, 'Alive to the glory of God: A key insight into St. Irenaeus', *Theological Studies*, 49, 283–297.

Donagan, A.: 1977, *A Theory of Morality*, University of Chicago Press, Chicago.

Engelhardt, H. T.: 1991, *Bioethics and Secular Humanism: The Search for a Common Morality*, SCM Press, London.

Irenaeus: 1979 *Against Heresies*, 4, 20, 7 in A. Roberts, J. Donaldson (eds.), *The Ante-Nicene Fathers*, Vol. 1, Wm. Eerdmans, Grand Rapids, Michigan.

BENEDICT M. ASHLEY O.P.

DOMINION OR STEWARDSHIP?:
THEOLOGICAL REFLECTIONS

I. BIBLICAL PRINCIPLES

Human puzzlement over the advantages and risks of technology is not new. The ancient Jews lived between the two oldest centers of human civilization, the cities of Egypt and of Mesopotamia. They attributed the discovery of technology to the evil descendants of Cain (Gn 4).[1] The building of the Tower of Babel (Gn 11: 1–9), they thought, caused the division of human languages and nations. God through the prophet Samuel warned them of the dire consequences when they asked for a king that they might rival other nations in technological, economic, and military power (1 Sm 8: 1–22; 1 Kgs 12 ff.; McCarter, 1980, 153–162; Jones, 1984, 1, pp. 247–256).

These biblical themes all show how aware the Jews were of the ethical dilemmas that advancing technology brings. Yet the Biblical attitude toward technology is not wholly negative, since the good use of technology is attributed to the "spirit of God" which works "in wisdom, knowledge and skill in every kind of craft" (Ex. 31: 2–3; cf. Sir 38; cf. also Westermann, 1974, p. 343). Hence, the Torah (the "Old Law") provided many detailed moral instructions to regulate the use of the relatively simple technologies of the time. These laws established principles which the Oral Law elaborated in the Talmud and which the countless rabbinic *responsa* of later Judaism have applied to all the details of technology in its development even down to the "high tech" of our own day (Neusner, 1984, pp. 1–27; Rosner, 1986).

Christians are not bound by the Mosaic Law as such (Sanders, 1978, pp. 103–126), but the teaching of Jesus does oblige them to the original *order of creation*, to the natural law as that has been elevated by grace to lead us to life in the Triune God. This is why the first chapters of the *Book of Genesis* with their symbolic account of that original order serve as an introduction and hermeneutic key to the Torah. According to that narrative, humankind has been created in God's "image and likeness" to share in God's *dominion* over creation, that wise, loving care by which he

85

K.Wm. Wildes (ed.), Birth, Suffering and Death, 85–106.
© 1992 *Kluwer Academic Publishers. Printed in the Netherlands.*

guides to their perfection and fulfillment whatever he has made.[2] Unlike the Mesopotamian and Greek myths which portrayed humans as made to be the slaves of gods jealous of their power, *Genesis* portrays a generous God who invites us to be his co-workers.[3]

Such cooperation implies that God has also endowed humanity with spiritual intelligence and will. Though we are made from matter, like other earthly creatures, God has breathed into us a spiritual life of self-consciousness and freedom. The somewhat abstract statements of Chapter 1 of *Genesis* are fleshed out in the vivid narrative of Adam and Eve in Chapter 2. God created this pair, placed them in the ideal environment of the Garden of Eden, yet gave them a task to perform. They were not to be hunters, but non-violent vegetarians who shed no blood (Gn 1: 29–30). They were to "take care of" the Garden, i.e., to protect the ideal environment given them by God, yet they were also to "cultivate" it, that is, work with God to bring it to still further perfection (Gn 2: 15).[4] To do this they had to understand God's purposes for each of his creatures, and this insight into their natures is indicated by Adam's naming the animals (Gn 2: 19–20).

Yet God also warned Adam and Eve that their co-dominion with him could not be absolute. All the garden was for their use, even the tree of immortal life, except for the tree of the "knowledge of good and evil" (Gn 2: 16–17). The serpent deceitfully explained this exception to Eve, "God knows well that the moment you eat of it your eyes will be opened and you will be like gods who know what is good and what is bad" (Gn 3: 5). Jesus exposed this lie in his Parable of the Two Sons (Lk 15: 11–32), proclaiming that God desires nothing of us but that we should share his blessed life. Adam and Eve, however, yielded to the serpent's illusion and were no longer content to cooperate with their Creator, but claimed to determine for themselves, apart from God, their own standards of right and wrong. In the New Testament Jesus reinforced and advanced this teaching of *Genesis*. First, he preached the coming of the Kingdom in which the New Adam, though he is a Spirit-anointed king (Messiah), is also a servant, (Phil 2: 7)[5]; and insisted that this servanthood applied to all his followers. "Whoever would be first among you must be your slave" (Mt 20: 25–28). Second, he worked great miracles of healing, of commanding the forces of nature, and of feeding the poor, which imply that we humans are empowered by God to regain the original rational dominion of Adam over nature, over disease, over poverty and want, if we will only use this power for service not domination.[6] Finally, in the

Parable of the Talents Jesus taught us that we will be responsible to God for the use of the gifts he has given us. It is not enough merely to return these gifts, but we must use them creatively (Mt 25: 14–30; Lk 19: 11–27). In the Last Judgment the criterion between salvation and damnation will be whether the plantiff has or has not served all other human beings as if they were Jesus himself (Mt 25: 31–46).

Thus the Biblical principles for an ethics of technology can be summed up as follows: (1) In creating us intelligent and free, God has given us a share in his dominion over the world and our own lives; but (2) this co-dominion is a *stewardship* which is to be exercised in cooperation with God in the completion of his creation according to his wise plan for our own happiness; and (3) therefore, human technology is not an absolute but a relative dominion under the guidance of God's loving wisdom and care and empowered by his grace.[7]

II. NATURE, ART, AND GRACE

Christian theologians early had the task of translating the biblical metaphors of God's dominion and humanity's stewardship into the abstract philosophical language of the Greeks. For the Greeks the natural world was the product of the art (*techne*, in the broad sense of technology) of the gods, and as such reflected the divine purposes.[8] Hence it must be used by humans only to further these embodied purposes. Therefore, humans are subject in their behavior to a "natural law" intrinsic to the very structure of natural things, including the human being as an organism, an ensouled body (Simon, 1965; Arntz, 1966, pp. 87–120; Luijpen, 1967, pp. 91–111; Finnis, 1980; Battaglia, 1981; Rhonheimer, 1987). Thus Greek ethics, in the main, was built on the principle that human behavior must be conformed to the intrinsic *teleology* or purposefulness of things (Ashley, 1967; 1973, pp. 267–284) .

Conformity to natural law for humans, however, was not for the Greeks merely blind instinct as for brute animals, but both an intelligent concord with nature and a transcendence of it. The concordance was expressed by the saying, "Art imitates nature" (Aristotle, *Physics*, II, c.2, 194a 22; Thomas Aquinas, S.C.G., II, c.75; W. Tatarkiewicz, 1973); while the transcendence was expressed by, "Art perfects nature."[9] Art derives its principles from nature, but through human invention it extends these principles to carry nature beyond itself. These two maxims, "Art imitates nature" and "Art perfects nature" thus provided Christian theologians with a way to translate the Biblical notions of "dominion" and "stewardship".

A third saying was added to these Greek ones by the medieval theologians to give the first two a specifically Christian character: "Grace perfects nature" or "Grace presupposes nature." (Stoeckle, 1962). This meant that God through the Incarnation has begun to repair the Creation fallen into ruin through the sin of angels and human beings and not only does he restore the world but has chosen to elevate it by grace to a share in the divine life itself, to deify it.[10] Hence as nature ought not to be wiped-out by human art, so also nothing that is human, both from nature and from art, is obliterated but perfected by grace. For Christians, therefore, as Vatican II in *The Church in the Modern World* has declared,[11] technology becomes an instrument of grace in the redemption of the world when it is concordant with God's purposes, when, so to speak, it perfects nature by "imitating" God.

III. SCIENCE AND NATURE

Today, however, the Biblical view of technology expressed in these Greek terms by theologians does not easily translate into the language of a scientific and technological age.[12] The principal area of conflict between theologians and scientists today is not, as many suppose, *creationism*, which is a problem only for fundamentalists.[13] The real barrier between contemporary theology and science is the notion of *nature*. "Nature," in the Greek understanding traditionally accepted by Catholic theology, implies teleology and since Newton, at least, scientists tend to think in non-teleological, i.e., mechanist terms. They explain the world in terms of matter moved by *purposeless forces*.

Yet, historians of science have demonstrated that the origins of this rejection of teleology by science, were not from within science itself, but was due to the triumph of Nominalism in the theological faculties of the late medieval universities (Weisheipl, 1959; Ashley, 1958, pp. 157–164). It is necessary, therefore, to ask whether this rejection is really scientifically necessary or even possible.

Since it is empirically verifiable that living organisms in their parts and as totalities develop themselves and perform characteristic activities such as feeding and reproduction to meet innate requirements of survival and thus are purposeful structures, biologists admit they exhibit "teleonomy", but deny they exhibit teleology.[14] Biologists argue that since this observable adaptation of living structures to the functions necessary for the organisms' survival can be explained as the result of the Neo-Darwinian natural selection of chance mutations through adaptation to the environment, any reference to teleological explanations would introduce an unnecessary and non-empirical factor outlawed by sound scientific method. Yet to admit into science the notion of "adaptation for survival", that is, of the relation of the structure to function and function to the very existence of the organism, is to admit the notion of the relation of "directedness" which is all that philosophers and theologians mean by the term "teleology".[15] Thus "teleonomy" and "teleology" are not rival explanations but two *correlative* aspects of a single, empirically observable phenomenon, that of adaptive functions considered on the one hand as to their origin in natural selection, and on the other precisely as adaptive.

Some would grant the intrinsic teleology of organisms, but deny it of inanimate natural entities. Admittedly goal-directed activity is more evident in living than non-living things. Yet the sciences of physics and chemistry would not be possible without the distinction between natural, chance, and artificial processes. Natural processes arise from forces inherent in physical objects prior to human manipulation and thus differ from artificial processes which always presuppose them. Technology has to use natural processes; it does not create *ex nihilo*.

Moreover, natural processes are also prior to chance events, which result from some unique concurrence of natural processes. Thus we call a process natural, and therefore subject to scientific investigation, because it is not a unique event resulting from chance, but instead regularly reoccurs, can be repeatedly observed, and then expressed by a natural law. Processes which regularly reoccur, however, can be identified only because they produce uniform results, and are thus predetermined to a goal, i.e., because they are teleological. Chance events are non-teleological. Artificial processes are teleological, but not intrinsically teleological, since their directedness is imposed by man on nature.

Yet even if we grant a teleology intrinsic to organisms and even to inanimate natural units, can we speak of a teleology intrinsic to the environment? Our earthly environment, like the human organism, is also a system, the ecosystem, but unlike an organism, it is not an *unum per se*, a substantial entity, but an inter-related collectivity of substantial entities (Owen, 1974; Peacocke, 1979, pp. 255–318; Joranson and Butigan, 1984; Moltmann, 1985, pp. 20–52).

An ecosystem does not, therefore, have an intrinsic teleology in the same sense as do the parts of an organism or the organism as a whole. Yet it is one of the discoveries of ecology that the inter-relations of the various organisms and inorganic bodies that compose an ecosystem, although not substantial, are something more than merely accidental. The entities (or at least many of them) depend for their very existence and survival on the system as a whole. For example, the correlation between the anatomy of an insect and the structure of the flowers from which it gathers honey and which in the process it pollinates – this mutual adaptation – is clearly teleological. This mutual dependence of the various entities that make up our earthly environment is scientifically verifiable (Barrow and Tipler, 1986).

Thus we can conclude that in an important sense (although not in the same way as is an organism) the terrestrial ecosystem is intrinsically teleological. What is special to the relation of humanity to its environment, of course, is that by our intelligence we exercise a dominion over the other members of the system and even to a degree the system as a whole, a dominion that is increasingly effective. This freedom proper to human nature, along with our materiality by which we are subject to chance, is the reason we are historical beings. Yet human historicity does not, as is often thought today, obliterate universal human nature, since, as we have seen, chance and freedom *presuppose* nature.

IV. SCIENCE AND ETHICS

If it is granted that science can contribute to the study of the intrinsic teleology of our environment in relation to the intrinsic teleology of the human person, we can now move to the ethical aspects of the technological application of science. Catholic theology has traditionally defended the notion of a "natural moral law", but there are many versions of what this term means. Moreover, today theologians who use it must be ready to defend their own versions against the many philosophical attacks to which all such theories have been exposed. I have made a defense of my own version elsewhere, and there is no space to summarize it here.[16] Whatever theory of the natural law a theologian adopts as philosophically defensible she or he must face up to two questions which cannot be answered without reference to the empirical sciences: (1) Can we empirically discover in the human species a common nature, invariant through cultural variations, which is teleological, so that it will make sense to say that certain kinds of behavior are "good" because they contribute to making the human being fully what it was made to be, i.e., what it "ought" to be?[17] (2) Can we empirically verify a teleological relation between our earthly environment and human nature such that it makes sense to say that certain man-made modifications of this environment are "good" for the human species and others are "bad"?[18]

The second of these questions is subordinate to the first, since if we cannot determine what is good for human persons, it will be meaningless to ask how humans should use or modify the environment. Is it not illogical to fight to conserve the ecological balance as if it were teleological, i.e., intrinsically purposeful, while at the same time failing to affirm an intrinsic purposefulness in the human structure, and attributing ethical norms purely to cultural convention? Equally absurd is the extravagantly altruistic notion, put forward by some enthusiastic "Greens", that we should preserve the environment for the environment's sake, not for ours, even to our disadvantage.[19]

Thus, if the ecological movement, which maintains that the teleological structure of the environment can be scientifically studied and technologically preserved and enhanced in the service of humanity, is a reasonable enterprise; then must it not also be acknowledged that an ethics based on the notion of "natural law", i.e., of an intrinsic teleology of human nature, can be objectively developed and applied? In Biblical terms this means that the human moral code can and should reflect not arbitrary human willfulness but the order of the world established by its Creator. One can reasonably defend such a teleological ethics without claiming that the order of creation is easily ascertained, or that principles so derived can be applied easily and certainly.

Questions of value, therefore, are not to be relegated to the realm of human subjectivity, but are open to objective rational debate to which scientific discoveries are directly relevant. Science can sharpen our understanding of natural law and natural law ethics can guide the technological application of science to human living.

But how could the empirical methods of science possibly contribute to the establishment of ethical norms? Is it not true that the classical ethical systems such as those of Aristotle or Kant have been developed independently of modern science? Must we admit that these traditional norms are open to falsification by modern scientific discoveries? Certainly it is fallacious to argue, as is so often done, that because Aristotle's natural science was rendered obsolete by Galileo and that of Newton (on whom

Kant relied) by Einstein, therefore Aristotelian or Kantian ethics are obsolete. Thomas Kuhn's famous theory of "scientific revolutions through paradigm shifts" (Kuhn, 1970; Gutting, 1980) does not negate the fundamental continuity of the development of science from Aristotle to Einstein traced by historians (Wallace, 1974, 2, pp. 238 ff.; Cohen, 1980).[20]

Einstein actually retrieved a more Aristotelian notion of space and time than Newton's. Likewise ethics today continues to built on the foundations laid by Aristotle or Kant. We can look to science therefore, not to create an ethics *ex nihilo*, but to assist in refining traditional ethics. The more science reveals to us about the structure and function of creatures, the more accurate will be our understanding of their teleology and hence of the natural law which furnishes the foundation of ethics. If art is to imitate nature and perfect it, the better we know nature the better will be our work of imitating and perfecting. The better also will be our stewardship of God's gifts.

The Biblical and conciliar teaching which I have just expounded can in a more philosophical manner be formulated as a simple principle: *Human beings are morally obliged to use and to modify the natural environment and their own bodies in accordance with their intrinsic teleology.* If God's purposes are knowable (at least in part and with the probability to be expected in practical matters) through the *intrinsic* teleology of creatures and if this teleology can be manifested by scientific investigations, then an area of common interest for science and theology is opened up. It is this common ground which Catholic moral theology has generally defended as the "natural moral law" however diversely explicated.

To illustrate and test this principle I will take two examples, the first from ecology, the second from bioethics, to exemplify the type of ethical argument which I believe is appropriate to each. In neither case will I attempt a detailed analysis, but only an illustrative outline.

V. ENDANGERED SPECIES

A prime concern of ecologists is the preservation of endangered species. According to the evolutionary reconstruction of the history of the earth, species arise from previous species and then disappear to make room for still newer species. Only a few species, usually in isolated niches of the environment, last for long. Why then is it a problem that the arrival of the human species is destroying other living species at an ever more rapid pace, increasing in our times to a holocaust?[21]

The reason usually given for alarm, is that this devastation of other life forms will so upset the ecological balance of the earth, that the human species also will be threatened with self-destruction. No doubt there is reason for alarm if this alteration of the environment proceeds heedlessly and without planning. Is it not possible, however, that we can make plans so that as we displace other species we may create an artificial environment, a man-made ecological system even more suitable for human life than the so-called natural environment that has predominated up until this century? Indeed as the human population increases and technology advances, is it not necessary for us to assume this control? Do we really need other animals than ourselves? Do we really need trees and flowers? Do we even need the sun and moon or the seasons if we can more successively control and use nuclear fusion as the source of all the energy we need?

These questions reveal, I think, that there is a more basic reason for preserving the natural environment than the riskiness of radically altering it. Would we really want to live in a purely artificial environment, such as might be constructed on the moon – an environment without trees or flowers, birds or fish? Our need for a natural environment is not merely practical, it is also esthetic, or more even more profoundly, contemplative. Biblical ethics, as well as that of Plato and Aristotle, holds that the ultimate fulfillment of human nature, its teleology, is the contemplation of God mirrored in the cosmos and best known to us by analogy to our human intellectuality (Aristotle, *De Anima*, III, 4, 429b sq.; *N.E.*, X, 7, 117a12 sq.; *Meta.*, XII, 1074b 15 sq.; Thomas Aquinas, *S.C.G.*, II, 1–4 and *S.T.*, I–II, q. 3, a.8).[22]

Hence, our need for the natural environment is not merely to supply us with energy, light, air, food, water, and a place to walk; but to provide us with the mirror in which we see God, both to delight our senses and to enrich our minds through scientific investigation. In short we have an ethical obligation to preserve our natural environment so that artists may paint it and scientists explore it for our delight. To destroy a species is to lose an irreplaceable masterpiece.

One may object that the new technology of genetic reconstruction offers hope that someday we may get control of the very process of evolution and thus replace the present environment not just with parking lots, airports, and shopping malls, but with a new living ecosystem of far more wonderful life-forms than we have today. I concede this is a real possibility, but a possibility that finally faces us with an oft neglected truth that human "creativity" is not truly creation *ex nihilo* but imitation (the Aristotelian *mimesis*).[23] As stewards of God's creation, we are "co-creators" in that we can perfect nature, but only by imitating it, by realizing in more detail what is already present in outline in nature. Perhaps we can "control" evolution, but only by understanding and employing the forces and potentialities of nature and getting our "creative ideas" from contemplating the forms it already has. When we lose sight of this essentially mimetic character of human art, as modern art tends to do today, we end in an empty minimalism of ideas and feeling. Similarly in technology we end with a environment which is either too polluted or too sterile for human life.

Thus the ecological movement is profoundly right in declaring that we must treat our planet like a garden, to be perfected, yes; but to be reduced to a wasteland out of which we will create a new world for ourselves, no. Our human goal is to know God, the Divine Artist, in his works. Our art is like that of the performer who enters into the vision of the composer by interpreting his composition and thus shares that vision and delight, but who remains a performer and interpreter not a composer.

VI. EUTHANASIA

Let us turn now from ecology to bioethics proper. A very controversial set of bioethical issues are those concerned with the obligation to treat dying or severely deteriorated persons and, more generally, with the human control over life and death. Some, of course, deny that it is ever moral to destroy any living thing; others restrict this to sentient things. The Fifth Commandment is "Thou shalt not kill" (Ex 20: 13) and *Genesis* seems to say that in the original design of God, men and even animals were vegetarians, since the permission to eat meat was only a concession to fallen humanity (Gn 1: 30; 2: 16; 9: 2–5). Yet the Old Law sanctions capital punishment and just wars (e.g. Dt. 19: 21–20: 1). Jesus on the contrary seems to have taught non-violence at least towards other human beings (Mt 6: 38–48), but Paul accepted law enforcement by the sword (Rm 13: 4).

Catholic Tradition has harmonized these Biblical teachings by holding that while humans may use plants and animals for any legitimate human purpose, they may not *directly* kill any innocent human being for any reason.[24] Yet the community may execute criminals to preserve the order of justice and the common good, and the community and its individual members may defend themselves against aggression even if this results in homicide as an unintended although foreseen effect. Furthermore, it has usually been held by Catholic moralists that one may sometimes allow persons to die of injuries, disease, or old age, when the only means available to maintain their lives exact too heavy a burden either on the victim himself or those who have the responsibility of care (Grisez and Boyle, 1979; Bernadine, 1988; Van Beeck, 1988, pp. 115–122; McCormick, 1989, pp. 369–388).

Why, in view of the various aforesaid qualifications of the commandment against killing, is it not permissible for intelligent and free human persons, knowing that death is inevitable at some time, to choose the most fitting time, and to kill themselves or permit others to do so? Are there not also situations in which it would be better for one human being to decide this for other sufferers who lack the competence or at least the courage to make this "death with dignity" decision for themselves?[25]

In the Catholic tradition the basic problem on whose answer all these other questions depend, has been whether suicide is sometimes licit, as pagan moralists taught and as seems to some to be the case in martyrdom. The veneration of the martyrs led to moralists making the distinction between indirect and direct killing, and later this distinction proved helpful in discussing the morality of war, abortion, and euthanasia (Finnis-Boyle-Grisez, 1987, pp. 297–322; Ashley, 1989; CDF 1974, 1980, 1987). As for direct suicide the answer commonly accepted by theologians was that to kill oneself contradicts the fact that life has been given us by God only in stewardship, to use in God's service but not to destroy. Some recent writers have criticized this argument on the grounds that it presupposes what it is supposed to prove, namely, that although God has given us intelligent, autonomous control over our lives, yet he has forbidden us to exercise this control to end our lives (Schüller, 1970).

No doubt it was because classical theologians anticipated similar objections that some of them, notably St.Thomas Aquinas (*S.T.*, II–II, q. 64, a.5)[26] bolstered this *argument from God's dominion* with two other arguments. The first is that as social animals we share in the common good to which we therefore owe our services and our persons, but by killing ourselves we deprive society of these goods to which it has a right in return for the good shared with us. Some, however, have questioned whether this *argument from the common good* really applies to suicide by someone who is no longer of service to society, perhaps indeed has become a burden to it.

The third argument is that suicide is contradictory to the fundamental human need to live; i.e., it is contradictory to the intrinsic teleology of human nature. It would seem that Aquinas in proposing this third *argument from intrinsic teleology* has made explicit a presupposition of the other two arguments without which they are inconclusive and even circular. It is because suicide contradicts the intrinsic good of human nature that it also contradicts the good of society, since society exists to aid the perfection of its members. Even when a member seems no longer useful to the community, and has even in some respects become a burden to it, such a "useless" member remains precious to society precisely because a community exists for the good of each and all its members.

Again, that God has made us stewards of our life yet has retained his own absolute dominion over its beginning and end we know not simply by revelation, but by the natural law which is simply an expression of the intrinsic teleology which God has given to human nature. To take our own life is to deny who we are, persons made to live, to guard and cultivate ourselves as living beings. In my opinion, therefore, the traditional argument against suicide, and consequently against all forms of euthanasia, remains valid and free of tautology. We know that our dominion over ourselves is that of stewardship not of autonomy when we understand the intrinsic teleology of our own natures, physical and spiritual. That stewardship demands the tender care of the dying and the alleviation of their pain, but it limits our claim to an absolute autonomy which would permit us to destroy innocent human life directly.

When we apply this general approach to the problems of bioethics and environmentalism, we get the following results. Every bioethical problem reduces to a question about the intrinsic teleology of the human person. This teleology must not be understood in a merely physicalist sense, but also it must not be understood dualistically.[27] To take a rather crass example, consider the discussion of homosexuality and the attitude to be taken toward it by the physician and the psychiatrist. It would be physicalistic simply to say that male homosexuality is unnatural because the teleology of the genital organs shows that the penis is adapted to the vagina and not other orifices in view of reproduction; but it would be dualistic simply to deny that it is unnatural on the grounds that the morality of physical acts depends wholly on the subjective spiritual meaning they have for the actors, not on their physical details.

Instead one could argue that homosexual actions are wrong because human sexuality, as a dimension of the total human person, has an intrinsic teleology that is not realized except in a male-female relationship of committed love consummated by using the bodies in a way conformed to the teleology of the genitals as reproductive. Thus the physical structure of a sexual act is morally significant not in isolation from the meaning of sexuality for the whole human person, but precisely as an act of the human person who is at once spiritual and physical.[28]

Another example can be found in the bioethical question about the obligation to use so-called "ordinary" or "extra-ordinary" means to maintain life in the severely deteriorated patient, such as one in the persistent vegetative state (AMA, 1986; AAN, 1986, pp. 125–127). To argue, as some do, that intervenous nutrition and hydration are always ordinary and obligatory if they are necessary to maintain life, on the grounds that to discontinue them is to kill the patient, or because life, even in this condition (Barry, 1986, pp. 498–471; May, pp. 203–210, NCCB Pro-Life, 1986) is still an inestimable value outweighing most burdens of care, is to forget that the obligation to take means to perserve life diminishes as the value of this life, measured in terms of its intrinsic teleology, diminishes. Human bodily life by its intrinsic teleology has its value from its service to activities of the whole human person, and especially to those activities which are specifically human, the spiritual activities of knowledge and free choice. When these activities become permanently more and more difficult or impossible, the corresponding obligation to perserve bodily life diminishes. That is why most moralists will admit that it is not obligatory to prolong life in the person who is actually dying if this becomes proportionately burdensome; and it seems to me that this holds also for such cases as the persistent vegetative state, even if one maintains that such a stable patient is not dying (O'Donnell, 1987; O'Rourke, 1988 a and b; Ashley and O'Rourke, 1989, pp. 374–386; O'Donnell, 1987).

Thus in this case as in all ethical dilemmas arising from technology the important thing is to establish intrinsic teleology as the ultimate measure of morality. This principle, philosophically coherent with empirical science, is theologically confirmed by the biblical teaching that God has created us in his image and given us a stewardship over his creation, a stewardship to be exercised creatively and harmoniously within the Creator's general purposes.

NOTES

[1] Claus Westermann, in his standard *Genesis 1: 11: A Commentary* (1974), 342-344, whose exegesis I have generally followed in this paper, accepts the view of Jean Paul Audet, "Le Revanche de Prométhée ou Le drame de la religion et de la culture," *Revue Biblique*, 73 (1966), 1–29, that the point of the biblical author is *not* that technology was the invention of the evil Kenites, but rather that this advance brought with it opportunities for evil. "The Cain and Abel narrative says that when people created by God live side-by-side in brotherhood there is at the same the possibility of killing. The song of Lamech indicates that the increased progress activated by the human potential increases the possibility of mutual destruction." (p. 337). (Cf. also Speiser, 1964; Plant, 1981).

[2] Westermann (1974, 147–160) reviews the complicated exegetical history of "image and likeness" (Gn 1: 26, 27; 5: 1; 9: 6; Ps. 8: 5–8) and concludes with Karl Barth that this phrase does not describe human nature, but God's purpose in creating us, namely, to be able to relate to God and communicate with him. The texts of Gn. 1 and of Ps. 8, however, explicitly and immediately connect the notion of "image" with the command to "multiply, fill the earth and sudue it," and only imply relationship in that God issues commands to Adam. Only in Gn 2 is mutual relationship more explicitated.

[3] "According to the Mesopotamian myths man was made to be the servant of the gods, to be a kind of breadwinner of his divine masters, to be the builder and caretaker of their sanctuaries. In the initial chapter of *Genesis* man was created to be the lord of the earth, the sea, and the air. The luminaries were created for the earth and the earth was created for man ... A certain degree of human dominion over creation is understood in the Babylonian account ... which charges man with the building of sanctuaries and the bringing of offerings. But in the first place, this is not explicitly stated. And in the second place, it is the dominion or authority of a *servant*, not of a lord. Each account stresses an entirely different aspect of man's place in nature" Alexander Heidel, *The Babylonian Genesis*, (1963, 121). A similar contrast with the Greek account of human creation in Hesiod's *Theogony* and *Works and Days* and in Aeschylus' *Prometheus Bound* is made by Audet (1966).

[4] Joseph Fuchs (1987) has pointed out the danger of anthropomorphism in speaking of the human creature "working with God", yet himself speaks of the human person as "constituted by the Creator as dialogical and cooperative partner" (p. 47–48). Even the term "partner" hardly does justice to the infinitely different orders of the actions of Creator and creature.

[5] "Then comes the end, when he [Christ] hands over the kingdom to his God and Father ... so that God may be all in all" (I Cor 15: 24, 28b).

[6] The miracles of Jesus should not be understood as making technology unnecessary, but as signs to us show us that by God's grace we can use technology to overcome many human ills. For example, liberation theology interprets the miracles of the feeding of the multitudes (Mk 6: 34–44; 8: 1–9) as a summons to feed the poor by properly distributing the abundance produced by modern technology.

[7] Recent discussion centers on the need for greater emphasis on a theology of creation as the context for a theology of redemption (Scheffczyk, 1970, Hendry, 1972). Macquarrie (1971) denies God "needs" creation, but argues for a "mutual" relation of

God and creation. Reumann (1973), as a Lutheran, defends the primacy of redemption and restricts the "new creation" to the redeemed community. Young (1976) is critical of Reumann, but allows the possibility of four different Christians attitudes toward creation: (1) the *transcendental* favoring "alienation" or withdrawal from the world (Karl Barth); (2) the *ontological* favoring "coalition" or identification with the world (Paul Tillich); the *existential* favoring "innovation" (Rudolf Bultmann); and the *eschatological* favoring "revolution" (Jürgen Moltmann). Bernhard W. Anderson, *Creation versus Chaos* (1987) attributes cosmic evil to the free choice of creatures and deals at length with the ecological problem.

8 Aristotle, *De Partibus Animalium*, I, 5, 644b 23–645a 37 develops this idea to show that biology, although it deals with earthly, short-lived beings is worthy of study although it does not deal, like astronomy, with heavenly, imperishable beings.

9 St. Thomas Aquinas combines the two principles neatly when he writes, "Art imitates nature and supplies the defect of nature in those things in which nature fails", Sent. IV, d.42, q.2, a.1 c.

10 The term "deification" (*theosis*) of the human person by grace, much favored by the theology of the Eastern Church, does not imply that Christians will be absorbed into God in a pantheistic manner, but that they will become "partakers in the divine nature" (*theias koinonoi physeos*) (2 Pt 1: 4).

11 "Far from considering the conquests of human genius and courage as opposed to God's power as if humanity sets itself up as a rival to the creator, Christians ought to be convinced that the achievements of the human race are a sign of God's greatness and the fulfillment of his mysterious design. With an increase in human power comes a broadening of responsibility on the part of individuals and communities: there is no question then, of the Christian message inhibiting human beings from building up the world or making them disinterested in the good of their fellows: on the contrary it is an incentive to do these very things." (Vatican II, GS # 34, 1965), (I have modified the translation to inclusive language).

12 See Leeuwen (1964), for a discussion of Christianity's role in developing a scientific technology. White (1967, pp. 1203–1207) accused *Genesis* 1–2 of causing the ecological crisis by teaching our unlimited domination of nature. Among the numerous replies were those by Froelich, (1970), Freudenstein, (1970), Santmire, (1970) (who admits that Church has indirectly encouraged anti-ecology), Fackre, (1971), Sherrel (ed., 1971), Jonas (1972), Richardson, (1972), Basney, (1973) and Hendry, (1980).

13 On the recent "creation science" controversy in the U.S.A. see Frye, 1983; Gilkey, 1985. The Bible seeks the ultimate cause of the very existence of the cosmos and of the spiritual element in humanity; while science only studies existing material processes and modestly admits that the ultimate question of "Why does anything at all exist?" is beyond its ken. Even if science asserts, as neo-Darwinianism does (Monod, 1972), that evolution is ultimately a matter of chance, yet God can use, not only natural law, but also both free actions and chance events to perfect his creation. For current discussion of this topic between scientists and Catholic philosophers, see McMullin (1985).

14 "Teleonomy" (goal-lawfulness) is used by some evolutionary biologists to indicate functionality or adaptation without any implication of "purpose".

[15] The use of the term "directiveness" was proposed and strongly defended in biology by E. S. Russell, *The Directiveness of Organic Activities* (Cambridge: Cambridge University Press, 1945).

[16] For recent reviews of controversies see Battaglia, 1981, Budziszewski, 1986, Hittinger, 1987; Goffrey Sayre-McCord, 1988. For my own discussion see *Theologies of the Body*, pp. 356–482 with bibliographic notes.

[17] On the famous Humean problem of the "is" and the "ought" which has plagued so much of modern metaethcis see the essays in Philippa Foot (1967), especially W. K. Frankena's essay,"The Naturalistic Fallacy" showing this is not a fallacy, but a dispute between cognivist (realist) and non-cognivist (emotivist) ethics. This debate has broken out again recently, (cf. McNaughton, 1988; Boyd, 1988; and John Finnis (1980), pp. 36–48). That this problem may be a result of misreading Hume see Alasdair MacIntyre, (1978, pp. 109–124).

[18] I have difficulties about the distinction between "good-bad" and "right-wrong" used by some ethicists today, but this is not the place to discuss that point. I follow common non-technical usage here according to which "good" = "beneficial" and "bad" = "harmful" according to teleological conformity or discomfority.

[19] Thus Peter Singer (1977) argues for rights of animals on a par with human rights. Some today even speak of "speciesism" as a sin similar to racism and sexism. On the other hand the International Network for Religion and Animals, which publishes a *Network News*, North Wales, PA and Silver Spring, MD, with more theological balance, promotes an "ecumenical" concern for animal welfare.

[20] Kuhn considerably softened his original thesis in subsequent work (Musgrave, 1980). Cohen (1980) shows that behind the "paradigm shifts" are micro-"transformations of ideas" which leave the substantial achievements of previous theories intact. My point here – perhaps too obvious – is only that "paradigm shifts" in science do not *necessarily* render obsolete theories of ethics generated by older scientific views.

[21] For summaries of the issues see the special number of *Managing Planet Earth*, (1989), especially Clark, pp. 46–57 and Wilson, pp. 108–117.

[22] See also St.Augustine's *Confessions*, Bk IX., c.10 and the whole tradition of Platonic Christian Theology described in Ashley, (1985), pp. 103–147. O'Connell (1969) shows that the exegesis of Gn 1 in *Confessions* XI–XIII is integral to the whole work's theme of the return of the soul to God, because the soul returns to God through the contemplation of creation.

[23] For a discussion of the theories of human creativity and my reasons for preferring a modified theory of *mimesis* see my *Theologies of the Body*, pp. 312–319.

[24] An effect is "directly intended" if an agent chooses to produce it, while effects which he does not choose to produce, but which he foresees may in the circumstances follow upon what he directly intends are said to be "indirectly intended." The term "innocent" (Latin *non nocens*, harmless) refers not to moral innocence, but to someone not engaged in an aggressive act. Thomas Aquinas (S. Th., II–II, q. 64, a. 6, 7) distinguished between the direct intention of an executioner to kill a criminal, and the indirect intention to prevent an act of aggression, by one who foresees that in this attempt he may kill the aggressor, although he tries to avoid this by doing the least damage necessary. Hence the concrete norm is "Direct killing of the innocent is

always forbidden." Killing in a just war was traditionally justified as punishment authorized by public authority of a criminal, or, (since the criminality of the enemy soldier was dubious) as an indirectly intended result of an attempt to prevent his aggressive act. Consequently, the laws of war forbid killing a soldier who has been rendered harmless ("innocent").

[25] Answers to these questions may depend on the more general issue of the methodology of moral judgement. Catholic moralists have generally held there are some absolute concrete negative moral norms because certain acts by their very nature are contradictory to the basic teleology of human nature. Hence, these are in all circumstances and for whatever motive performed *objectively* morally evil (*intrinsice malum*) and thus *exceptionless*. Thus Josef Fuchs (1965, p. 123) wrote, "For example, it can never happen that a prohibition of a direct destruction of unborn life – a principle of the natural law – could cease to be an absolute demand even in a difficult concrete situation, or out of charitable consideration for a mother and her family." The controversy over *Humanae Vitae* (1968), however, provoked an effort to revise this fundamental principle by a new methodology of moral judgement called by its critics (of whom I am one) "Proportionalism" because of its exclusive reliance on what is called the "principle of preference" or "of proportionate reason". Surprisingly, Fr. Fuchs himself led this revision by what still remains one of its clearest statements (Fuchs, 1970 [1979]; see also the important articles of Knauer and Janssens in the same volume, and Schüller, 1985, pp. 165–192). This position has been extensively criticized as both impracticable and self-contradictory; for the literature see Grisez, (1983, 1, pp. 141–172). The risks of this proportionalist method are evident from the fact that some, for example Maguire (1984), think it justifies euthanasia in certain current circumstances, while others such as Schüller, (1985) and McCormick (1989) reject suicide as forbidden by a *virtually* exceptionless concrete norm, because they feel that only in very rare cases would its values outweigh its disvalues.

[26] Aquinas' arguments were developed extensively by Francisco de Vitoria in his *Relectio de Homicidio* ([1587] 1960) and Cardinal de Lugo in his *Disputatio de Homicidio* ([1642] 1869).

[27] Thus Charles E. Curran (1980, 76) writes, "... the primary problem with the official hierarchical teaching is its physicalism or biologism. The physical act must always be present, and no one can interfere with the physical or biological aspect for any reason whatsoever. The physical becomes absolutized. Most revisionist Catholic theologians today will argue that for the good of the person it is legitimate at times to interfere with the physical structure of the act. Note that it is precisely in questions of sexual morality that Catholic teaching has absolutized the physical and identified the physical with the truly human or moral aspect. For example, there has always existed an important distinction between killing and murder, since murder is the morally condemned act, whereas killing is the physical act which is not always wrong. However, artificial contraception understood as a physical act is said to be always and everywhere wrong." This caricatures the "official hierarchical teaching" on human sexuality which, far from "absolutizing the physical," emphasizes the "dignity of the person" as a whole (cf. Lawler, Boyle, and May, 1985) to which the body and its physical acts are intrinsic and essential.

[28] This is my understanding of the ethical basis of the "Letter to Bishops of the

Catholic Church on the Pastoral Care of Homosexual Persons" (CDF, 1986). For comments on that document see G. Ramick and Furey (1987), and Ashley (1987), 105–111.

BIBLIOGRAPHY

Books

Anderson, B.: 1987, *Creation versus Chaos*, Fortress Press, Philadelphia.

Aristotle: 1957, *De Anima*, W. S. Hett (trans.), Harvard University Press, Cambridge, MA.

Aristotle: 1961, *De Partibus Animalium*, A. L. Peck (trans.), Harvard University Press, Cambridge, MA.

Aristotle: 1982, *Nicomachean Ethics*, H. Rackham (trans.), Harvard University Press, Cambridge, MA.

Aristotle: 1935, *Metaphysics*, Harvard University Press, Cambridge, MA.

Ashley, B.: 1985, *Theologies of the Body: Humanist and Christian*, Catholic Health Association, St. Louis.

Ashley, B. and O'Rourke, K.: 1989, *Healthcare Ethics: A Theological Analysis*, Catholic Health Association of the United States, 3rd ed, St. Louis.

Augustine of Hippo: 1953, *Confessions*, V. J. Bourke (trans.), Fathers of the Church, vol. 21, New York.

Barbour, I. G.: 1990, *Religion in an Age of Science*, The Gifford Lectures, 1989–1991, vol. 1, Harper and Row, San Francisco.

Barry, C.: 1986, *Human Nature*, Humanities Press International, Atlantic Highlands, New Jersey.

Battaglia, A.: 1981, *Toward a Reformulation of Natural Law*, Seabury, New York.

Bernadin, *et al.*: 1988, *The Consistent Ethics of Life*, (ed.) by Thomas G. Feuchtmann, Sheed and Ward, Kansas City, MO.

Budziszewski, J.: 1986, *The Resurrection of Nature*, Cornell University, Ithaca, New York.

Congregation for the Doctrine of the Faith: 1974, *Declaration on procured abortion*, *Osservatore Romano*, Dec. 5, 1974.

Congregation for the Doctrine of the Faith: 1980, *Declaration on euthanasia*, *Origins*, 10, 154–157.

Congregation for the Doctrine of the Faith: 1987, *Instruction on respect for human life in its origin and on the dignity of procreation*, *Origins* 16 (40) 697–709.

Cohen, I. B.: 1980, *The Newtonian Revolution: With Illustrations of the Transformation of Scientific Ideas*, Cambridge University Press, Cambridge, MA.

Crowe, M. B.: 1977, *The Changing Profile of the Natural Law*, Martinus Nijhoff, The Hague.

Curran, C. E.: 1988, *Tensions in Moral Theology*, Notre Dame University Press, Notre Dame, Indiana.

Curran, C. E. and McCormick, R. A.: 1979, *Readings in Moral Theology, No. 1. Moral Norms and Catholic Tradition*, Paulist Press, New York.

D'Entreves, A. P.: 1964, *Natural Law*, Humanities Press, Atlantic Highlands, New

Jersey.

Donagan, A.: 1977, *The Theory of Morality*, University of Chicago Press, Chicago.

Dyson, F. J.: 1988, *Infinite in All Directions*, Gifford Lectures, 1985, Haper and Row, San Francisco.

Fackre, G.: 1979, *Ecology Crisis: God's Creation and Man's Pollution*, Concordia Publishing House, St. Louis.

Finnis, J.: 1980, *Natural Law and Natural Rights*, Clarendon Press, Oxford.

Finnis, J., Boyle, J. M., and Grisez, G.: 1987, *Nuclear Deterrance, Morality and Realism*, Clarendon Press, Oxford.

Foot, P.: 1988, *Theories of Ethics*, Oxford University Press, Oxford.

Frye, R. M.: 1983, *Is God a Creationist?: The Religious Case Against Creation-Science*, Charles Scribner's Sons, New York.

Fuchs, J.: 1965, *Natural Law: A Theological Investigation*, Sheed and Ward, New York.

Gilkey, L.: 1985, *Creationism On Trial*, Winston Press, Minneapolis, MN.

Gramick, J. and Furey, P. (eds.): 1987, *The Vatican and Homosexuality*, Crossroad, New York.

Grisez, G. G.: 1983, *The Way of the Lord Jesus*, Franciscan Herald Press, Chicago.

Grisez, G. G. and Boyle, J. M.: 1979, *Life and Death with Liberty and Justice: A Contribution to the Euthanasia Debate*, University of Notre Dame Press, Notre Dame, IN.

Gutting, G.: 1980, *Paradigms and Revolutions: Appraisals and applications of Thomas Kuhn's philosophy of science*, University of Notre Dame Press, Norte Dame, IN.

Heidel, A.: 1963, *The Babylonian Genesis*, University of Chicago Press, 2nd ed., Chicago.

Hendry, G. S.: 1980, *Theology of Nature*, Westminister Press, Philadelphia.

Jones, G. H.: 1984, *1 and 2 Kings*, New Century Commentary, Wm. B. Eerdmans, Grand Rapids.

Joranson, P. N. and Butigan, K. (eds.): 1984, *Cry of the Environment: Rebuilding the Christian Creation Tradition*, The Center for Ethics and Public Policy, Santa Fe, NM, Bear and Co., Berkeley, CA.

Kuhn, T.: 1970, *The Structure of Scientific Revolutions*, 2nd ed., University of Chicago Press, Chicago.

Lawler, R., Boyle, J., and May, W.: 1985, *Catholic Sexual Ethics: A Summary, Explanation, and Defense*, OSV Press, Huntington, IN.

Leeuwen, A.: 1964, *Christianity in World History*, Edinburgh House, London.

Lugo, J.: 1869, *Tractatus de Justitia et Jure Disputationes Scholasticae et Morales*, Dis. X, vol. 6, 36–56, "De Homicidio", J.B. Fournials (ed.), Vives, Paris.

Luijpen, W. A.: 1967, *Phenomenology of Natural Law*, Duquesne Philosophical Series 22, Duquesne University Press, Pittsburgh.

McCarter, P. K.: 1989, *I Samuel, Anchor Bible*, Doubleday, Garden City, NY.

MacIntyre, A.: 1981, *After Virtue: A Study in Moral Theory*, University of Notre Dame Press, Notre Dame, IN.

MacIntyre, A.: 1978, *Against the Self-Images of the Age*, Notre Dame University Press, Notre Dame, IN.

McMullin, E.: 1985, *Evolution and Creation*, Notre Dame University Press, Notre Dame, IN.

McNaughton, D.: 1988, *Moral Vision*, Basil Blackwell, Oxford.

Maguire, D.: 1984, *Death by Choice*, Doubleday, Garden City, NY.

Moltmann, J.: 1985, *God in Creation*, Harper and Row, San Francisco.

Monod, J.: 1972, *Chance and Necessity*, Collins, London.

Neusner, J.:, *Invitation to the Talmud*, Harper and Row, 2nd ed., San Francisco.

O'Connell, R. J.: 1969, *St. Augustine's Confessions: The Odyssey of the Soul*, Belknapp Press of Harvard University, Cambridge.

O'Rourke, K. D.: 1988, *Development of Church Teaching on Prolonging Life*, Catholic Health Association of America, St. Louis.

Owens, D. J.: 1974, *What is Ecology?*, Oxford Press, London.

Peacocke, A. R.: 1979, *Creation and the World of Science*, The Bampton Lectures, Clarendon Press, Oxford.

Plant, W. G.: 1981, *The Torah: A Modern Commentary*, Union of American Hebrew Congregations, New York.

Reumann, J.: 1973, *Creation and the New Creation*, Augsburg Publishing House, Minneapolis.

Rhonheimer, M.: 1987, *Natur als Grundlage der Moral: die personale Struktur des Naturgesetzes bei Thomas von Aquin: eine teleologischer Ethik*, Tyrolia Verlag, Innsbruck.

Santmire, B. E.: 1979, *Brother Earth: Nature, God, and Ecology in a Time of Crisis*, Nelson, New York.

Sayre-McCord, G. (ed.): 1988, *Essays on Moral Realism*, Cornell University Press, Ithaca, NY.

Scheffczyk, L.: 1970, *Creation and Providence*, Herder and Herder, New York. Ed. *Scientific American*, 261, September 1989, *Managing Planet Earth*.

Sherrel, R. E. (ed.): 1971, *Ecology: Crisis and New Vision*, John Knox Press, Richard, VA.

Simon, Y.: 1965, *The Tradition of Natural Law: A Philosopher's Reflections*, Fordham University Press, New York.

Singer, P.: 1977, *Animal Liberation: A New Ethics for our Treatment of Animals*, Avon, New York.

Speiser, E. A.: 1964, *Genesis, Anchor Bible*, Doubleday, Garden City, NY.

Stoeckle, B.: 1962, *Gratia supponit naturam*, Herder, Rome.

Strauss, L.: 1953, *Natural Right and History*, University of Chicago Press, Chicago.

Thomas Aquinas, St.: 1951, *Aristotle's De Anima with the version of William of Morkbeke and the Commentary of St.Thomas Aquinas*, Kenelm Foster and Sylvester Humphries (trans.), Yale University Press, New Haven, CT.

Thomas Aquinas, St.: 1961, *Commentary on the Metaphysics of Aristotle*, John P. Rowan (trans.), Henry Regnery Co., Chicago.

Thomas Aquinas, St.: 1964, *Commentary on the Nicomachean Ethics of Aristotle*, C.I. Litzinger (trans.), Henry Regnery Co., Chicago.

Thomas Aquinas, St.: 1956, *On the Truth of the Catholic Faith (Summa Contra Gentiles)*, Anton C. Pegis *et al.* (trans.), Hanover House, 1956, Garden City, NY.

Thomas Aquinas, St.: 1974, *Scriptum super libros Sententiarum*, M. F. Moos ed.,

Lethielleux, Paris.
Thomas Aquinas, St.: 1964, *Summa Theologicae*, Latin and English translation, McGraw Hill, New York.
Vitoria, Francisco de, *Obras*, Teofilo Ordanz, O. P., ed., *Relectiones Theologiae* [1587], Madrid, Biblioteca de Autores Christianos, 1960, "De Homicidio," pp. 1070–1130.
Weisheipl, J. A.: 1959, *The Development of Physical Theory in the Middles Ages*, Sheed and Ward, New York.
Westermann, C.: 1974, *Genesis 1–11: A Commentary*, Augsburg Publishing House, Minneapolis.
Young, N.: 1976, *Creator, Creation, and Faith*, Westminister Press, Philadelphia.

Articles

American Medical Association, Report of the Judicial Council: 1986, 'Treatment of patients in irreversible coma'.
American Academy of Neurology; 1986, 'Care and management of persistent vegetative state patients', *Neurology*, 39, 125–127.
Arntz, J. T. C.: 1966, 'Die entwicklung des naturrectlichen denkens innerhalb des thomismus', in Franz Bockle, (ed.), *Das Naturrecht im Disput*, Dusseldorf, Patmos Verlag, pp. 87–120.
Ashley, B. M.: 1987, 'Compassion and sexual orientation,' in Grammick, J. and Furey, P. (eds.), *The Vatican and Homosexuality*, Crossroad, New York, pp. 105–111.
Ashley, B. M.: 1990, 'Contemporary understandings of personhood', in *25th Anniversary of Vatican II: A Look Back and a Look Ahead*, Pope John Center, Braintree, Ma.
Audet, J. P.: 1966, 'Le revanche de prométhée ou le drame de la religion et de la culture', *Revue Biblique*, 73, 1–29.
Barry, R.: 1986, 'Withholding and withdrawing treatment', *Journal of the American Medical Association* 256 (4) 498–471.
Basney, L.: 1973, 'Ecology and the spiritual concept of the master', *Christians Scholars Review*, 49–50.
Boyd, R. N.: 1988, 'How to be a moral realist', in Sayre-McCord, pp. 256–181.
Clark, W. C.: 1989, 'Managing planet earth', *Scientific American*, 261, 46–57.
Frankena, W. K.: 1967, 'The Naturalistic Fallacy', in Foot.
Freudenstein, E. G.: 1970, 'Ecology and the Jewish tradition', *Judaism*, 19, 406–414.
Froelich, K.: 1970, 'The ecology of creation', *Theology Today*, 27, 263–276.
Fuchs, J.: 1979, 'The absoluteness of moral terms', in C. E. Curran and R. A. McCormick, S. J., (eds.) *Readings in Moral Theology, No. 1. Moral Norms and Catholic Tradition*, Paulist Press, New York, 8.
Fuchs, J.: 1987, 'Our image of god and innerworldly behavior', in *Christian Morality: The Word Becomes Flesh*, Brian McNeill (ed.), Georgetown University Press, Washington, DC, 28–49.
Jonas, H.: 1972, 'Technology and responsibility' in James Robinson (ed.), *Religion and the Humanizing of Man*, Council on the Study of Religion, New York, 1–19.

Hendry, G. S.: 1972, 'The eclipse of creation', *Theology Today*, 406.

Lonergan, B.: 1974, 'The transition from a classicist world-view to historical mindedness' in *A Second Collection*, W. F. J. Ryan and B. J. Tyrell (eds.), Westminister Press, Philadelphia, 1–9.

Macquarrie, J.: 1971, 'Creation and environment', *Expository Times*, 4–9.

May, W. E., *et al.*: 1987, 'Feeding and hydrating the permanently unconscious and other vulnerable persons', *Issues in Law and Medicine*, 3(3), 203–210.

Musgrave, A. E.: 1980, 'Kuhn's second thoughts', in Gutting, 39–53.

O'Donnell, T.: 1987, 'Comment', *Medical-Moral Newsletter* 24(2).

O'Rourke, K. D.: 1986, 'The AMA statement on tube feeding: An ethical analysis', *America*, 155(15), 321–328.

Richardson, C.: 1972, 'A christian approach to ecology', *Religion in Life*, 41, 462–479.

Schüller, B.: 1985, 'The double effect in Catholic thought: A reevalution' in *Doing Evil to Achieve Good*, Richard A. McCormick, S. J., and Paul Ramsey (eds), University Press of America, Lanham, MD, 165–192.

Tatarkiewicz, W.: 1973, 'Mimesis' in *Dictionary of the History of Ideas*, Phillip P. Wiener (ed.), Charles Scribner's Sons, New York, 3, 225–230.

U. S. National Conference of Catholic Bishops, Committee for Pro-Life Activities: 1986, 'Statement on uniform rights of the terminally ill act', *Origins* 16 (12) 222–224.

Van Beeck, F. J.: 1988, 'Weaknesses in the consistent ethics of life?: Some systematic theological observations', in Bernadin, 115–122.

White, L.: 1967, 'The historical roots of our ecological crisis', *Science*, 155, 1203–7.

Wilson, E. O.: 1989, 'Threats to Biodiversity', *Scientific American*, 261, 108–117.

DIANA BADER O.P.

SHARING RESPONSIBILITY AT THE EDGES OF LIFE

INTRODUCTION

A. Recent Cases

(1) In New York a two-day-old infant was diagnosed as clinically brain dead. A week later when the members of the ICU staff explained to the parents in Spanish that "the infant was clinically and irreversibly brain dead and that his heart and lungs functioned only with the aid of the respirator and medication," the parents, who are Jehovah Witnesses, refused to acknowledge the infant's death and requested that the hospital continue providing life-supporting medical therapy. The Trial court ruled that the hospital could remove the life supports from the brain dead infant, but delayed implementation of the order so that parents could either appeal the decision or arrange a transfer to another institution. The parents, praying for a miracle, insisted on continued life support for the infant, stating that "If they take him off the respirator they will be committing murder" (McIntyre, 1989).

(2) When a 67-year-old man with a medical history of myocardial infarctions, chronic obstructive pulmonary disease and arteriosclerotic heart disease had a poor recovery from major surgery for colon cancer, the attending physician and nurses found themselves in the center of a dispute as to who should make decisions for the man: his out-of-town daughters from a previous marriage or the woman friend with whom he had made his home for the last ten years? The daughters were adamant that everything should be done for the father; the woman friend who had been with the patient for most of his hospitalization asked that he be made comfortable, but that no heroic measures be taken.

B. Challenges

Cases like these reflect tensions that can accompany end-of-life decisions. A unilateral decision by one person which is not supported by others who

107

K.Wm. Wildes (ed.), Birth, Suffering and Death, 107–126.
© 1992 *Kluwer Academic Publishers. Printed in the Netherlands.*

must implement the decision is a difficult solution to the conflict. The sharing of responsibility in these situations could relieve the tensions. There are, however, a number of circumstances that make sharing decision making responsibility difficult: ambivalence regarding death, misunderstanding about roles and responsibilities in making decisions about dying, tensions in the relationships that surround the dying person, uncertainty about the parameters and limits of individual autonomy in the use – or abuse – of medical treatment, and disagreement about the weight to be given to the dictates of religious faith in the dying process.

These difficulties are compounded by medical practices that deny or ignore the appropriateness of sharing responsibility for life-death decisions. For example, the tradition of medical paternalism supports the physician as the lone decision-maker for treatment decisions, and the one solely responsible for the well-being of the patient. At the same time, the community dimension of dying has been cast into the shadow by the attention given to life-saving technology. In the past, death was a community event. Those closest to the patient ministered in a variety of ways: watching and praying with the patient, listening and talking, laughing and weeping. In solidarity, a close community bore the painful experience together. Today, because of the medicalization of the healthcare setting, death is more often regarded as a failure of medical science. The dying find themselves isolated from human warmth and compassion in institutions, cut off from access to human presence by technology which dominates the institutional setting in which most deaths occur.

Personal attitudes toward death can likewise be a source of tension. While some dread death, others see it is as the fitting conclusion to the events of life. For still others, it is a welcome release from suffering and diminishment. Many can appreciate death as a mystery, and they seek to neither hasten or delay its arrival. Often, death itself is not feared as much as the isolation, misunderstanding and overbearing technology that may surround dying.

The task of caring for those at the edges of life is to accompany the dying, to help them to approach their last act with faith, dignity and serenity. Treating the physical, psychosocial, and spiritual needs of the dying is not within the capability of any one individual or group. Rather we must look to multidisciplinary teams who can share the responsibility for creating an environment of humane dying.

The search for clear norms in caring for the dying is made difficult by

some of the pressures that bear, directly or indirectly, on the circumstances of dying today:
- *Modern medical technology which imposes*, along with awesome benefits, overwhelming burdens on those who use and provide it – physical pain, emotional stress, financial pressures, ethical tensions, etc.
- *Uncertainty of diagnosis and prognosis*, which makes it difficult to predict the course of a patient's illness, and the length and quality of life with or without treatment.
- *Patients' rights movements* with emphasis on patient autonomy and the implications for doctor-patient relationships.
- *Recognition of the professional status of nurses* with a need to recognize their appropriate authority and responsibility as members of the healthcare team.
- *Increasingly active role, especially in the U.S., of the law and the courts* in resolving fundamental conflicts over the use or foregoing of life-sustaining technology.

These factors are playing out in a world in which an increasing incidence of dementia and painful financial constraints bedevil the best efforts to make sound, ethically responsible decisions in end-of-life situations.

C. Questions

If dying is to be more than a failed technological occurrence, it will call forth a diversity of resources and responses which translate into shared responsibility. This is dictated by our interdependence as members of a community and by the range of the needs to be met.

I will attempt to probe the meaning of shared responsibility by considering:
- The key relationships in end-of-life situations.
- The dimensions of shared responsibility at the end of life – *Who* is expected to share responsibility?.
- Obstacles to successful sharing of responsibility for the dying.
- Some practical implications of sharing responsibility in decision-making for the dying.

TOWARD HUMANE DYING: SHARING THE RESPONSIBILITY

A. *Christian Perspective*

Religious faith casts a particular light on the meaning of shared responsibility. Christian faith is rooted in belief in an ultimate power, a personal God incarnated in time and place in Jesus Christ. It is nourished by the symbols and stories that help to interpret the events of human history in which the presence of God is encountered. The Christian affirms that

"... all human life is the gift of God ... endowed with the capacities for knowledge, freedom and personal relationships, we are called in community to realize the divine purpose of living which is to love God and one another ..." (Methodist-Roman Catholic, 1989)

To love God and one another is the effect of the individual person's tendency toward ultimate unity, in which it finds its fulfillment. In Christian theology, the tendency toward unity creates an inclination toward ever more intimate union, with ourselves, with others, and with God. Union with God is sought in virtue of the radical dependency on the Creator, who is the fullness of all being. Human love is also and necessarily a tendency toward union with other human persons, distinguished in space and time. "The agent of our union and unity with ourselves and with God, love is thus the principle of our communion with others" (Gilleman, pp. 132).

Because of our personal need, human love tends to seek the other for personal enrichment. Only when the satisfaction of personal need becomes an absolute end and not a phase of communion does love become destructively egotistic. Love of neighbor when it is appreciated as communion causes a consciousness of the other and an ability to reach out beyond personal self-interest to the good of the other.

Love is truly an ecstasy which causes us to go forth from carnal self, with which we are easily tempted to identify ourselves because our sensibility is so infected by egoism. This is why love normally appears as an abnegation, a sacrificing of our temporal interests, and hence as gratuitous and disinterested – an attempt to attain, in its own way, the perfect gratuity of divine love (Gilleman, pp. 143–144).

Women and men in their radical tendency toward unity in love form a community of persons who are radically interdependent throughout life – for their origin, survival and continuing nurture.

The human vocation includes a special privilege and responsibility of sharing in the continuing work of creation: helping to form a world in which relationships of love find behavioral expression in communities of mutual concern and responsibility. However, evil, suffering and death are realities of the world we know

In the face of the ultimate mystery of why humans suffer and die ... we experience God always seeking to turn suffering and death into wholeness and life. These realities call us to witness to God's presence in the midst of suffering by sharing compassionately in the tasks of healing the sick and comforting the dying .... Only (in the resurrection) ... will the mystery of suffering and death find its complete answer. Until then holy living and holy dying means mutual support among pilgrims on the way (Methodist-Roman Catholic, 1989)

In the Christian schema charity, as love of God, transforms life through virtuous action. Charity is the virtue that orders the moral life. Because of the orderly nature of love, some objects of love take precedence over others. Thus, God is loved first and foremost; all others are loved in God (Aquinas, *Summa Theologica*, II–II, 25, 1). While charity inclines toward identification or union with the other, justice is the virtue which provides the moral norms governing relationships among individuals and classes of persons. It is important to emphasize that love of neighbor is a central requirement of justice.

Justice, based on recognition of human dignity, structures relationships among persons. Human dignity is protected through fundamental rights – claims to resources and services that help to assure the attainment of life's goals. At the end of life, certain rights become especially critical to a patient: the right to respectful treatment of one's person, to participation in decisions affecting one's care, the right to appropriate holistic care. While these rights imply obligations for the caregivers, they also carry reciprocal obligations for the patient: to respond, within one's resources, to the ministrations of those charged with attending the dying. The virtue of justice challenges our tendency to isolation, to feel secure in the satisfaction of our own individualistic needs, and to settle complacently with our own achievements. In the setting where one of us is ending his or her life, it calls for deep respect for one another and generosity in uniting as a community to contribute our complementary gifts that make possible a humane dying.

For Christians, therefore, lively religious faith will mean attending to one another, as individuals and as a community, when death begins to cast its shadow over a life. Dying persons and those caring for them will experience the end of life as sacramental, that is, as a moment in which the love and hope of the community signify and re-create the saving action of Jesus' death and resurrection extended to all who would receive it.

The particularities of mutual care and responsibility for one another in dying and in grieving will be considered now in the context of our contemporary experience of dying.

B. Goals of Care and Treatment

While care of the terminally ill has always been a concern of medical and nursing professions, the development of modern medical technology has overshadowed the dying person as the subject of our attention. With the focus on cure, diagnostic and therapeutic technologies have been generally directed toward those who have some reasonable hope of recovery. Thanks to the work of Dr. Cicely Saunders and the Hospice movement, the resources of modern medicine are being reclaimed for terminally ill and dying persons, and the patient is resituated at the center of care.

The goal of professional healing is the well-being of the patient, achieved through attention to the physical, mental, social, and spiritual needs of the dying person. Appropriate pain management to relieve physical pain; skillful interventions to facilitate the expression of denial, anger, depression, and other emotions which constitute mental pain; supportive services to allay guilt and sadness over unfulfilled social commitments; and sensitive pastoral attention to religious needs – all are aspects of the dying patient's well-being and goals of the terminal care.

C. Relationships in End-of-Life Situations

The basis of shared responsibility is found in the relationships that exist among patients, families and caregivers. What is the nature of the various relationships? Why are certain relationships given pre-eminence in caring for persons who are dying?

In his treatise on Charity Aquinas (*Summa Theologica*, II–II, 23–46) grounds on love the ordering of relationships to God and within the human community. First, charity-love implies benevolence, wishing well to the other. From benevolence flows beneficence; the act by which the will effectuates that which it wills (*Summa Theologica*, II–II, 23, 1; 31, 1).

Beneficence is a special act of charity. In its general notion it includes doing good to all. Beyond the general duty to all humankind, there is a special duty of beneficence that arises from one person's connectedness to another. As Aquinas says:

Now one man's nearness to another may be measured in reference to the various matters in which men are engaged together; ... and various benefits should be conferred in various ways according to these various fellowships; because we ought in preference to bestow on each one such benefits as pertain to the matter in which, speaking absolutely, he is most closely joined to us (*Summa Theologica*, II–II, 31,3).

Love admits of degrees, based on the connection that one person has to another. There is always an obligation to wish well to all people, but those to whom we are more closely connected have a stronger claim on our love, for example, those connected to us by kinship or citizenship (*Summa Theologica*, II–II, 26, 7).

The order of love can be further specified with regard to beneficiaries and benefactors. While there is a sense in which one's benefactors by their good works evoke love, those who receive beneficence are to be loved more. Why? Because the beneficiary becomes in a sense the handiwork of the benefactor and thus a natural object of love. Also, we tend to love more those in whom we see our own good. Those who serve others see the reflection of their own good in the ones who are served and thus are inclined to love the recipients (*Summa Theologica*, II–II, 26, 12).

Love will find formal expression in a number of virtues, one of which is mercy. Aquinas quoting Augustine characterizes mercy as "heartfelt sympathy for another's distress, impelling us to succor him if we can" (*Summa Theologica*, II–II, 30,1). Grief over another's distress is a moral attitude that prompts one to care for those who have reached the end of mortal life and require the special ministrations of kin and professionals.

The insights of Aquinas can be helpful in arguing the nature of and reason for the particular relationships that exist in end-of-life situations. The natural order of charity establishes the primacy of the family and mutual familial obligations, in benevolence and beneficence, to attend to the needs of the loved one who suffers and approaches death. Insofar as it can be said that the practice of "medicine arises in a universal human need that transcends the physician's idiosyncratic definition of its boundaries" (Pellegrino, 1983, p. 168), the need of the patient and the power (knowledge, skill, experience, compassion) of the physician ground the relationship. Healthcare professionals – physicians and all who collaborate with him/her – assume special obligations in love, benevolence and mercy to place their compassion and skills at the service of the sick and dying.

The behavior that characterizes relationships in the health care setting has been clarified – in fact, to a great extent, legitimated – by invoking certain images, metaphors and analogies. Metaphors for roles in the health care setting are drawn from a variety of contexts: family, church, business, war, etc. The metaphors traditionally used to illuminate or legitimate the role of the professional – notably the doctor – in health care include: father, priest, contractor, technician, captain, partner, friend. Correlative roles of the patient range from the role of a child to that of an equal partner. Conflict arises when parties see themselves according to different metaphors: for example, when a patient who regards himself as a partner in the health care enterprise encounters a physician who regards herself as having a parental relationship to the patient.

While the various metaphors are not mutually exclusive, and more than one may be operative in the way a professional conducts him/herself, the paternal image has dominated the practice of medicine in the Western world. Paternalism can be defined as "a refusal to accept or to acquiesce in another person's wishes, choices, and actions for that person's own benefit" (Childress, 1982, p. 13). Certain features of the paternal role are prominent in health care: first, the father's motives, intentions, and actions are assumed to be benevolent, aimed at his children's welfare; second, the father makes all or some decisions regarding their welfare rather than letting them make these decisions. The paternalistic approach continues to be justified by the assumption that the professional is acting on someone's behalf, although not necessarily at the other's behest.

Paternalism has been accepted by both partners in the doctor-patient relationship. Paternalism is widespread in health care not simply because beneficence tends to become paternalistic or because professionals desire power. To a great extent, health care professionals are paternalistic in response to social expectations. "Paternalism is not merely assumed, it is assigned" (Childress, 1982, p. 46).

The exercise of paternalism has been justified by the ethical principle of beneficence, that is, the ethical obligation to prevent harm to others and to secure their benefit. Dedication to beneficence as a norm has been a given in the health professions. Beneficence in its richest meaning is an act of love of neighbor, creating an ethic of love or care that is basically oriented toward benefiting the neighbor.

Because beneficence in its various forms may become paternalistic, love needs to be constrained by the principle of respect for persons, identifying with the projects and goals of another, and respecting the choices the other makes because they are his/her choices. Autonomy is one aspect of respecting persons as independent ends in themselves. The principle of respect for persons requires that we construe autonomy as a constraint upon our pursuit of goals for ourselves or for others. It does not require that we view autonomy as a goal or as an ideal... It is possible to respect others' wishes, choices, and actions in that they constrain and limit our pursuit of goals..." (Childress, 1982, p. 66).

The Christian virtue of justice, which regulates relationships among persons, can help to prevent or resolve tensions that may arise between the requirements of beneficence and the requirements of autonomy. When beneficence as love and autonomy as respect structure the relationships between patient and caregivers, there will be partnership or covenant, with all parties willingly assuming rights and obligations.

Ideally, sharing responsibility will be an expression of love and respect, helping to create a climate of trust and openness that encourages effective communication among all parties.

D. Dimensions of Shared Responsibility

When charity exists, creating the dynamic of union among members of a community, and justice is operative in relationships among individuals and classes of persons, the practical meaning of shared responsibility can be illustrated on a number of levels. First, the community: because of our inherently social nature, it is important to view the dimensions of shared responsibility from the perspective of human life in community. Second, individuals who comprise the community: all have particular gifts, competencies and tasks that together make life within the community possible. Third, society: the larger context which by its institutional structures and processes should assure the rights that protect human dignity.

Community: Sharing responsibility at the end of life will reflect a style of living in which relationships and interdependence among members of the community are valued and nurtured. In contrast to a spirit of in-dividualism in which self-conviction and self-direction isolate people from one another, the emphasis on community helps to convert a group from an aggregate of individuals pursuing self-interests to an interdependent community of mutual support. When physicians, nurses, chaplains, social workers and others see themselves as part of a community of care in which each person makes a specialized contribution, the pressure of decisions and their consequences is shared. It becomes appropriate to consult with others, to share information, to seek support, to challenge decisions, etc., without diminishing one's own role and contribution. This type of relationship is important today when the degree of specialization in healthcare disciplines often isolates individual practitioners from one another and from their patients. In a christian view of community the work of the health professions calls for partnership sustained by loyalty and trust.

A community, because of the diversity within it, can find creative ways to encourage sharing of responsibility. Such as:
- Being a catalyst for collaboration between groups – the parish, school, hospital, etc.
- Engaging the services of agencies and organizations that have outreach programs for the sick, elderly, and dying to provide education on aging, suffering, death; bereavement counselling, legal counsel, transportation, respite services.
- Promoting a spirituality that would provide a framework of hope and meaning in which to cope with suffering and dying.
- Developing and exemplifying the virtue of hospitality – providing emotional support and physical relief, not only to patients, but also to professional and family caregivers. Hospitality extends to accompanying the dying and those attending the dying in a faithful and loving way when curing is no longer possible (Gula, 1959).

Individual: Individual members of the community will be challenged to develop the virtues of loyalty, trust, courage and benevolence that make the sharing of responsibility possible. These virtues will manifest themselves in the different roles individuals take.
1. *Patient*: Respect for self that motivates efforts to take reasonable care of one's health and avoid undue risk and harm; confidence and trust in caregivers; readiness to cooperate and comply with care plans; accountability for decisions and actions that affect outcomes of treatment; and willingness to be an active participant in the communication processes necessary in sharing responsibility.
2. *Family*: Understanding and acceptance of the diminishments and

losses that accompany terminal illness; familial support of the dying loved one and of other bereaved members of the family; readiness to serve as compassionate and responsible surrogates for incapacitated family members; courage to assume an advocacy role when the best interests of the patient require it; availability and accessibility for the consultative processes that accompany life-death decisions; respect for all participants in the care setting – other family members, professionals, etc.

3. *Physicians*: Dedication to patient well-being, by maximizing benefits and minimizing risks and harms; acceding to the patient's request not to prolong life, but using medical resources when there is a good chance of providing an extension of life that will have the quality of life the patient seeks; readiness and ability to enhance patient autonomy by providing relevant information on diagnosis, prognosis, and treatment alternatives; facilitating the patient's process of understanding by active listening; assuming the role of patient advocate when the patient's interests are at risk; sharing authority and trust with other members of the health care team by soliciting information and encouraging participation in decision-making.

4. *Nurses*: Helping the patient to deal with the diminishments and losses of illness; encouraging the patient and family in their efforts to compensate for functional losses and limitations; advocating for the patient by offering other members of the health care team information, insight, perspectives on the patient's response to illness; assuming responsibility and authority in partnership with other caregivers.

5. *Social Workers, Chaplains, Other Allied Health Care Givers*: Attending to the distinct social, spiritual and mental needs of the ill patient; discovering resources appropriate to the individual's personal history and situation; helping to balance attention to physical symptoms with sensitivity to the psychological, social and spiritual needs of the person; offering specialized information and perspectives that will enhance the decision-making process when this serves the patient's needs; being available to families for specialized counseling, referral and support services.

6. *Attorneys, Risk Managers, Institutional Advocaters*: Offer special advice to support patients, families and caregivers and to relieve anxieties regarding legal obligations; discerning conflicts of interest

that may impede sound objective decision-making and/or create adversarial relationships among those who attend the dying patient.

All who care for the patient – doctors, nurses, other caregivers – will find ways to reaffirm the value of the person, and to counter the patient's temptation to feel unloved, of being an embarrassment or an inconvenience to those on whom he/she is dependent. Efforts to improve the overall sense of well-being in this way will help the dying person to accept this last act with dignity and serenity.

Society: Finally, a Christian understanding of sharing responsibility implies certain structures and processes within society. At the least it requires:
– The promotion within the professions of an ethos that builds on the dedication to healing and rewards respect for autonomy, both of patient and professional; that assigns priority to patient well-being over professional achievement and security (financial, legal, etc.); and that encourages sharing of authority among those with the responsibility and competence to exercise it.
– The promotion of legal and judicial processes that respect and tolerate ambiguity in end-of-life situations, and that refrain from unwarranted intrusions into the decision-making process, while defending the state's legitimate interests in the protection of human life, maintaining the standards of the medical profession, avoidance of euthanasia/suicide, and protection of the vulnerable (Cruzan, 1990).
– Equitable allocation of financial resources for health care based on need, with a view to steering a course between harmful privation for the underprivileged and extravagant overuse by the privileged; application of cost-benefit analysis to programs and services for persons at the end of life; financial accountability at all levels, creating a communal/societal consciousness of each person's role in striving for distributive justice.

E. Practical Implications: Obstacles and Suggestions for Practice

Practical problems can arise in the process of sharing responsibility when there is a conflict between the principle of beneficence and respect for autonomy. Practical questions and problems also arise when patients are decisionally-incapacitated. The model of shared responsibility can help resolve problems of communication, treatment decisions, and general decision-making

1. What must be emphasized at the outset is the fundamental and critical place of communication in sharing responsibility. Communication is more than the transmission of information. Founded on trust, effective communication involves an attitude of openness, appropriate self-revelation, and receptivity. It calls for particular skills in verbalizing thoughts, listening, interpreting, facilitating disclosure. Thus, the patient is encouraged to talk openly about death, and talking openly about death encourages and expands communication. In the process, the value of the person is affirmed. The willingness to expend the time required for good communication and to take the risks involved in active listening and self-disclosure will be, in part, the measure of one's willingness to share responsibility at the edges of life.

   More important than the debate about the limits of autonomy is the need for doctors and everyone else who is involved in the care of the terminally ill to communicate with their dying patients. Doctors need to be able to elicit the fears of dying patients and to discuss and answer those fears. They need to be able to discuss terminal care openly so that patients can see that they will not be abandoned and left helpless in the face of a terminal disease. (British Medical Association, 1988).

2. Some of the most difficult decisions involve the use of medical treatment at the end of life. Patients as well as caregivers may experience pressure to utilize all available treatments and life-prolonging interventions, regardless of their anticipated benefits. These pressures can arise from a variety of sources – fear of death, desire to avoid legal risk, economic incentives, need to maintain hope. While it is important to maintain hope in the face of death, authentic hope is founded on acceptance of the present reality with a firm conviction that life's larger goals can still be attained. Accepting the truth that further medical interventions offer little or no promise of cure can be an act of honest hope.

   There is no moral obligation to use medical interventions when the burdens of the intervention are disproportionate to the benefits to be expected (Bole; Wildes in this volume). Burdens include the pain and discomfort of the treatment itself, the indignities suffered in undergoing treatment, the economic strain on self or family, and the emotional burden to patient and/or family. The benefits are to be weighed not only in terms of extended life but also in relationship to the burden of the life itself that may result. As the Catholic Church teaches in the "Declaration on Euthanasia" (Vatican Congregation for the Doctrine of the Faith), due proportion is to be exercised in the use of remedies:

> Today it is very important to protect, at the moment of death, both the dignity of the human person and the Christian concept of life, against a technological attitude that threatens to become an abuse .... It is permissible to make do with the normal means that medicine can offer. Therefore one cannot impose on anyone the obligation to have recourse to a technique which is already in use but that carries a risk or is burdensome. Such a refusal is not the equivalent of suicide; on the contrary, it should be considered as an acceptance of the human condition, or a wish to avoid the application of a medical procedure disproportionate to the results that can be expected, or a desire not to impose excessive expense on the family or the community .... When inevitable death is imminent in spite of the means used, it is permitted in conscience to take the decision to refuse forms of treatment that would only secure a precarious and burdensome prolongation of life, so long as the normal care due to the sick person in similar cases is not interrupted.

The forms of treatment provided to a dying patient should therefore be adjusted to the condition of the patient and the prospects of medical benefit. Aggressive efforts to cure will give way to emphasis on palliative care and attention to the comfort needs of the patient when the hope of cure no longer exists. Far from abandoning the dying, such an approach is a loving act of "companying with" someone in their final journey.

3.   This perspective on the use of medical treatment options may not be shared by all those who are involved in end-of-life situations. The Congregation for the Doctrine of the Faith wrote that: "In the final analysis, it pertains to the conscience either of the sick person, or of those qualified to speak in the sick person's name, or of the doctors, to decide, in the light of moral obligations and of the various aspects of the case."

While individual autonomy is not an absolute, ordinarily the decisions of a patient who has decision-making capacity are to be honored. The fact that a patient's choices are not consonant with those of the family or professionals is not, in itself, relevant. The commitment to particular life goals based on values that have been espoused by an individual will influence one's choices in end-of-life situations. Only the dying person can fully assess the implications of personal goals and values for these choices.

The situation is more complex when a patient's request creates conflicts of conscience for others involved in implementing the request.

The request may, at one extreme, imply the refusal of standard interventions to alleviate or arrest symptoms; at the other extreme, it may call for heroic and expensive but futile efforts to forestall death. What may be at issue here is the principle of fidelity which creates positive obligations of beneficence in health care relationships. Mutual obligations and concomitant expectations are created when patient and physician enter a professional relationship for the care of the patient. Because the physician, in establishing a relationship with the patient, has made an explicit or implicit promise to seek the patient's best interests, the physician cannot without grave cause abandon the patient. The American Medical Association has written: "Once having undertaken a case, the physician should not neglect the patient, nor withdraw from the case without giving notice to the patient, the relatives, or responsible friends sufficiently long in advance of withdrawal to permit another medical attendant to be secured" (American Medical Association, 1986, p. 8).

The patient has an obligation to communicate openly with the physician, to provide the information necessary for sound medical judgment, and to cooperate in the care plan proposed by the physician. Certainly patients may disagree with the course of treatment advised by the physicians. When open dialogue fails to resolve a disagreement between patient and physician, the patient has options such as further consultations or engaging another physician. When the patient exercises autonomy in such a way as to reject or act outside the standards of treatment adhered to by the physician, the structure of the obligations in fidelity changes (Childress, 1982, pp. 341–342). The patient's right to continued treatment by this physician may be compromised; the physician may be justified in transferring the care of the patient to another medical professional. In caring for the patient, the physician retains his or her own moral agency. The physician does not become the slave of the patient, especially when ethical issues are concerned (Loewy, 1986, p. 100).

Conflict is not limited to that between patient and physician. Conflicts among professionals are not uncommon, especially in critical end-of-life situations. For example, the nurse who has attended a patient for long hours may feel better able to judge what is in the patient's best interests. Disagreement with the orders of attending or consulting physicians may produce a sense of responsibility to have the physician's order countermanded. There is no simple solution in such a situation. "Significant conflicts between health care professionals can be expected as long as there are major differences in degrees of participation in decision-making and in degrees of closeness and distance in the delivery of care. There will probably be political if not moral problems as long as some professionals make the decisions and order their implementation by other professionals who have not participated in the decision making .... There are no second order rules to enable professionals to resolve all the dilemmas created by conflicts between rules of fidelity and other principles and rules" (Childress, 1982, p. 348).

The commitment to patient autonomy does not mean that there is never room for a form of limited (weak) paternalism. In exceptional cases, the principle of respect for persons may warrant overriding the wishes or preferences of an individual who is, in some way, impaired and cannot act rationally and independently or cannot articulate an authentic course of action. Weak or limited paternalism is justified when: there is probability of harm; the intervention used is the least restrictive, the least humiliating, and the least insulting to the individual under the circumstances; and when there is procedural fairness. For example, it may be necessary in order to avoid serious physical, psychological, and social consequences of a major fall to impose physical restraints on a frail patient against his/her wishes. Or, it may be justifiable to temporarily assume decision-making for parents who are overwhelmed by grief at the birth of a seriously ill newborn. Such decisions should be implemented in a manner that respects the dignity and limited autonomy of the patient as far as possible

4.   The conditions for limited paternalism suggest the further dilemma posed by those whose decision-making capacity is impaired or totally lacking.

Decision-making capacity should not be equated with the legal standard of competency, which has different goals and criteria. The capacity for making health care decisions is not an all-or-nothing matter, but is situation specific, that is, more or less capacity is required according to the complexity of the decision to be made. Decisional capacity may admit of degrees in the same individual over different times and situations. Thus, judgments about capacity must be made for the here-and-now and be regularly assessed as new decisional demands are made.

The individual who lacks decision-making capacity has a need and right to have preferences, wishes, and values respected. This right may be protected in a number of ways.

First, prospectively one can execute advance directives, that is, specifying through written documents what treatments are to be provided at the end of life (living will); and designating a surrogate decision-maker to act on the individual's behalf when the latter is no longer capable of deciding (health care proxy). Whether advance directives are recognized as legally binding in a particular jurisdiction or not, they are a valuable guide to the patient's wishes and require respectful attention and sensitive interpretation.

Second, one can designate an appropriate decision-making surrogate: a person designated through an advance directive, or an immediate family member or close friend in a position to know what is in the best interest of the patient.

The role of a surrogate is especially important in an era when extended life-expectancy is accompanied by an increasing incidence of dementia. The surrogate becomes the voice of the dying patient, charged with making a decision that most closely approximates that of the patient. Ideally, this will be a substituted judgment: that is, executing the decision that had been expressed by the patient while competent. When no such prior decision had been made by the patient, the surrogate will rely on a best interest judgment: that is, deciding in light of all the objective and subjective factors, including the patient's personal values and goals, what is in the best interest of the patient.,

5.   Additional supports for the sharing of responsibility can be developed within the institutional setting.

Explicit policies on informed consent, use of life-sustaining treatment, surrogacy, etc., can clarify roles and responsibilities, empower those who must face difficult decisions, provide lines of accountability, and serve as valuable educational resources.

Institutional ethics committees can provide an interdisciplinary forum in which communication skills are enhanced and inter-professional rapport is developed as a committee addresses critical ethical issues and creates a resource for conflict resolution in exceptional situations when agreement cannot otherwise be reached.

Support groups, for families, to strengthen them through the dying process and in the bereavement period, and for professionals, to cope with the stresses of attending the dying person and in the emotional aftermath of death, can be of invaluable assistance.

CONCLUSION

The sharing of responsibility at the edges of life is not an end in itself, rather it suggests a process toward an end. It presumes agreement regarding the end to be sought, and willingness to work for that end even to the point of subordinating one's personal preferences when that is necessary to enable humane and compassionate dying. The sharing of responsibility will not automatically relieve the dying person's suffering, or eliminate the pain of loss experienced by loved ones, or prevent the conflict that can arise when a pluralism of experiences and values creates a clash. This approach, however, does offer the best hope for integrating the positive resources of all who participate in end-of-life situations and for creating incentives to focus on the well-being of the dying patient as a key concern.

Reflecting back to the two cases with which we opened this paper, a resolution of each is suggested by the preceding discussion. The presumption, based on their relationship to the clinically brain dead infant, favors the parents as the proper decision makers and their exercise of autonomy should be supported. However, when their demand for continued treatment, judged by prevailing medical standards, is unreasonable, it can be argued that the physician's obligation in fidelity and beneficence ceases. The patient/parent-physician relationship has changed and both parties have the option of terminating their relationship. The exercise of parental autonomy in this manner – acting contrary to established medical judgment – may limit the ways in which autonomy can be further exercised with regard to this situation. For example, other physicians may be unwilling to assume care of the infant; administrative leaders may intervene to enforce the standard of treatment (removing the respirator on brain dead patients); or a court order may be sought to replace the parents as legal guardians. But before such decisive steps are taken, every effort should be made to involve a representative group of caregivers in what will inevitably be a painful decision. The possibility of reaching a consensus will be much stronger when the parents are assisted not only by sound medical advice but also by the efforts of social and pastoral workers who may be able to address cultural, religious or other biases that complicate the parents' ability to understand the implications of the diagnosis and the advice that is given.

In the second case, physicians and nurses perplexed about the appropriate role of out-of-town daughters when decisions must be made for their decisionally incapacitated father should recognize the familial ties that establish a special relationship of benevolence within the family. Yet the presumption that favors the daughters' authority over that established by the ten-year relationship with his woman friend is questionable. To expand further on the order of charity discussed earlier, the friendship that originates from personal choice takes precedence over that of kinship. (Thomas Aquinas, II–II, 26, 8, ad 1). The father's choice of a life companion can be interpreted to reflect a relationship of benevolence, with both parties committed to the well-being of the other. The woman companion with whom the patient has freely chosen to make his home has a strong claim to the role of surrogate decision maker in this case. Indeed, practical wisdom suggests that her understanding of what the patient would want is as accurate and current as possible under the circumstances.

In summary, a commitment to shared responsibility at the edges of life will require work to develop:
– honest, trusting relationships in the health care setting;
– effective communication skills;
– ability to make well-reasoned burden-benefit judgments in the application of medical treatment;
– sound criteria for the rational use of health care resources.

As human beings, we all share the common passages of birth, life, and death. We are easily moved to multiply the joys of birth and life by sharing special moments with others. As christians let us be equally ready to alleviate the sorrow of dying by sharing responsibility among others. The alternative is isolation and abandonment of dying persons and those who attend them. That is a course that is not open to the Christian conscience.

BIBLIOGRAPHY

American Medical Association Council on Ethical and Judicial Affairs, *Current Opinions* – 1986: Chicago: American Medical Association.
British Medical Association: 1988, *The Euthanasia Report*, London.
Childress, J.F.: 1982, *Who Should Decide?*, Oxford University Press, New York.
Cruzan vs. MO Dept Health, *et al.*, V. 110 S. Ct., June 25, 1990 WL 84074 U.S.
Gilleman, G.: 1959, *The Primacy of Charity in Moral Theology*, trans. W.F. Ryan, S.J. and A. Vachon, S.J., Newman Press, Westminster, MD.
Gula, Richard: 1989, 'The virtuous response to euthanasia', *Health Progress*, 70, 24–27.
Loewy, E.: 1986, 'Physicians and patients: Moral agency in a pluralistic world', *Journal of Medical Humanities and Bioethics* (1), 57–68 cited in Ashley, B. M. and O'Rourke, K. D.: 1989: *Health Care Ethics*, 3rd ed. Catholic Health Association, St. Louis, MO.
McIntyre, R. L.: 1989, 'New York court sanctions hospital's removal of life supports

from brain dead "Infant Over Parents" objections', *Information Trends: Medicine, Law & Ethics*, 5, 1–4.

Methodist-Roman Catholic Agreed Statement: 1989, 'Holy living, holy dying', in *Origins*, 19, 241–248.

Pellegrino, E.: 1983, 'The healing relationship: The architectonics of clinical medicine', in Earl E. Shelp (ed.), *The Clinical Encounter: The Moral Fabric of the Patient-Physician Relationship*, E. Reidel Publishing Company, Boston.

Vatican Congregation for the Doctrine of the Faith: 1980, *Declaration on Euthanasia*, United States Catholic Conference, Washington, D.C.

Waymack, M., and Taler, George A.: 1988, *Medical Ethics and the Elderly*, Pluribus Press, Inc., Chicago.

PAUL SCHOTSMANS

WHEN THE DYING PERSON LOOKS ME IN THE FACE: AN ETHICS OF RESPONSIBILITY FOR DEALING WITH THE PROBLEM OF THE PATIENT IN A PERSISTENT VEGETATIVE STATE

I. PERSONALIST CRITERION FOR DISCERNING HUMAN DIGNITY

With the advance of medical technology the process of dying is often transferred to institutional settings. The purpose of my reflections is to present a Catholic, ethical framework for the care of the dying as an interhuman event. This anthropological-personalist approach implies that love, which forms the core of a Christian inspired, personalistic ethic, is not an accidental nor arbitrary invention of a particular religious revelation. On the contrary, love is rooted in the "nature" or createdness of humanity itself. The ethical task to love one's neighbor is our very essence. I can only dedicate myself actively and consciously to my fellow human beings and to the world because I am structured, according to my essence itself, as a "being-for-the-other-than-myself" (Burggraeve, 1988). Since the Enlightenment we have grown accustomed to placing autonomy at the center of ethical reflection. Relational philosophy, was (and is) considered as being irrational, dogmatically alienating, or contrary to emancipation. Autonomy does, however, not have the first nor the last word but it exists thanks to "creatural" solidarity and is a necessary condition for the fulfillment of this solidarity in a Christian perspective. In the relational approach of the human person,person is decentralized without being alienated, as opposed to the Western notion of autonomy which automatically connects relational responsibility and alienation. This becomes perfectly clear in the discussion of the care for the dying: the euthanasia movement is an expression of the Western notion of autonomy, while the relational-personalistic approach offers, in my view, the real openness for the promotion of the human person, adequately considered in himself and his relationships.

To be fully human in a Christian perspective, is both to exhibit and to participate in the wonder of a rich many-sidedness: to be human is to be rich in unity and originality (Autiero, this volume). From a Christian perspective originality is an empty concept if it does not include openness

127

K.Wm. Wildes (ed.), Birth, Suffering and Death, 127–143.
© 1992 *Kluwer Academic Publishers. Printed in the Netherlands.*

toward the other and if it does not involve cooperation with others for the expansion of a community. Responsible involvement is an important aspect of this interwoveness of personal self-development, relational encounter, and human solidarity. These are the three essential dimensions of the human person, adequately considered. According to this approach an act is morally good if it is beneficial to the human person adequately considered in himself and his relationship.

There are still two characteristics of the criterion of responsible involvement which help us understand the personal responsibility of the health care professional in concrete situations. In virtue of the historicity of the human person responsible involvement means that we must again and again reconsider which possibilities we have at our disposal in order to serve the promotion of the human person. This is a demand of a dynamic ethics which summons us to the imperative of what is better or more human according to its actualization becomes possible. In conjunction with this we must further, in our acts, respect the originality of all men and women as much as possible.

Before applying this ethical model to issues of death and dying such as the ethical problem of nutrition and hydration for the patient in a persistent vegetative state, let me first make clear that this general Christian ethical outline is quite different from some other proposals for ethical argumentation. It seems to me that an anthropology that is too restrictive and narrow will not adequately address issues of health care (Apostel *et al.*).

1. Utilitarianism and Deontology

Contemporary philosophical accounts of moral theory often loose the richness and complexity of human relationships by focusing on a narrow criterion, or set of criteria, in understanding anthropology and the moral dimensions of human life. The different forms of utilitarianism, for example, focus on the consequences of actions, rules, or preferences. While consequences are significant elements of human relationships, they do not capture the whole of our relationships to one another. Some acts have inherent ethical value despite their consequences. We refer to examples regarding professional secrecy: the betrayal of this secrecy can immediately provide many advantages. However, preserving it has an ethical value in itself not arising from its consequences. Thus the problem should be situated within the whole of human existence.

With this I have clearly posited that I want to stand at a good distance from the utilitarian model. The model of responsibility is equally distant from deontological theories. For these, the moral value of an act does not depend on its results, but from the qualities of the act seen in itself. How limited such an argumentation is, became clear in the discussion on amputation. Into the eighteenth century, mutilation was considered intrinsically evil. But by then surgery was sufficiently advanced that operations such as the amputation of a leg became possible in the case of gangrene. The general prohibition of mutilation was then provided with an exception: mutilation is intrinsically evil except when the giving up of a part of the body is necessary to save the whole. The same holds true of organ transplants which up until the 1940's were also considered as a form of mutilation. Most of the moralists who endorse the ethics of responsibility reason so: physical integrity is a great value and this will underline the prohibition of mutilation. But it is quite thinkable that this value must give way before another which is more important in the concrete circumstances: one's own life or the health of another human being.

2. The Principle of Double Effect

The temptation towards reductionism is also found, at times, in Christian moral theology. In many interpretations of the principle of double effect one finds a tendency towards physicalism. Confronted with the problem of nutrition and hydration for patients in persistent vegetative state, traditional Roman Catholic moral theology would invoke the principle of double effect as a method to deal with moral situations in which the outcome has more than one effect and the plural effects not all are good. As Kelly and Selling have made clear: the principle of double effect served as a framework for the application of physicalist criteria to medical ethical issues, enabling Catholic moralists to achieve universal applicability through precise cause-and-effect analysis (Kelly, 1950, 1951, 1957; Selling, 1980). The individual actions of physicians could be analyzed, dissected as it were, and a determination made as to their moral quality. Though the principle is well-known, it is useful to recall the exact formulation of its four conditions since other proposals of its wording and direction have been made. The principle of double effect, as the name itself implies, supposes that an action produces at least two effects. One of these effects is something good which may be legitimately intended;

the other is an evil that may not be intended. Granted the presupposition of good and evil effects, an action is permitted, according to the principle, if these conditions are fulfilled: the act itself must be morally good, or at least indifferent. Second, the agent may not positively will the bad effect but may permit it. If he could attain the good effect without the bad effect he should do so. The bad effect is sometimes said to be indirectly voluntary. Third, the good effect must flow from the action at least as immediately (in order of causality, though not necessarily in the order of time) as the bad effect. In other words, the good effect must be produced directly by the action, not by the bad effect. Otherwise the agent would be using a bad means to a good end, which is never allowed. Finally, the good effect must be sufficiently desirable to compensate for the allowing of the bad effect. In forming this decision many factors must be weighed and compared, with care and prudence proportionate to the importance of the case.

The first and second conditions of the principle served as a framework for the emphasis given to the physical goals and structures of the analyzed acts. The two conditions are really reducible to one another, and can be stated as one: the end does not justify the *physically specified* means. Moral quality was attributed to the act-in-itself on the basis of the position in the causal chain of the evil effect of the action and on this basis the final judgment was made. The evil effect was "direct", if it preceded the good effect as its cause, the evil effect was considered "indirect", if it lay outside the intention *of the act*. In the former case it was forbidden while in the latter the action was permitted. The other conditions of the principle had to be met as well, but in most of the issues of medical ethics the first two conditions determined the outcome.

It was this normative framework which enabled Catholic ethicists to make the well-known distinctions between active and direct, or passive and indirect, euthanasia. All the major manuals of Catholic medical ethics prior to the Second Vatican Council used this approach. This combination of normative and meta-ethical systems enabled Catholic moralists to arrive at precisely specified conclusions, based on physical cause-and-effect analyses, and backed up by a society whose authority could not be questioned. In a way which paralleled the approach of modern professional medicine, the "orthodox" solution could be demonstrated as "scientific", a term used by some authors. It could be applied regardless of situational flavor to all cases where the physical diagnosis was the same, could be explained in a special vocabulary and with precise kinds of specifications build up by specialists over the centuries, and could be proven by appeal to the only society ultimately qualified to make such decisions. The methodology was particularly apt for dealing with the kinds of issues which constituted the core of the discipline: individual actions of doctors and nurses and patients to deal medically with bodily ailments.

This kind of parallel to modern medicine proved, however, detrimental to Catholic medical ethics. It is not so much that Catholic moralists wanted to affirm what the doctors were doing; in many instances they rejected interventions proposed by the medical profession. The problem lies more in the professional and scientific ethos which Catholic medical ethics adopted and the kind of analysis which this ethos proposed as normative. However beneficial it might have been for medicine, this kind of ethos and analysis was ultimately unfit for a theological/philosophical ethical discipline. Health involves more than physical medical interventions. Its methodology was restrictive, since it largely ignored the theological principles on which it was supposedly founded and subordinated them to rigid methodological frameworks. The result was a normative absolutism which could ignore most of the contextual flavor of human life and reduce its analysis to physical and biological factors.

Since Vatican II, the emphasis on the external object as the primary font of morality has moved to the intentionality of the human person as this font. A personalist perspective acknowledges the imperfect nature of reality and places the burden on humankind to discover and to actualize the best proportion of good over evil by willed choice. In this perspective it is more accurate to place the moral weight of an action within the subject, the human person as free positer of moral action.

II. RELATIONAL-PERSONALIST APPROACH TO THE DYING:
AN APPLICATION

The Court of Law in Alkmaar (The Netherlands) observed in its ruling on euthanasia on May 10, 1983 that: "in ever wider circles, the right of self-determination with regard to the termination of life is becoming accepted". In its official report on euthanasia, the Dutch State Commission also bases itself on the right of self-determination in offering the opinion that euthanasia may be practiced with impunity if certain procedural rules are satisfied. With regard to this, Theo Beemer has accurately spoken of a withdrawal from a common search for the meaning of life (Beemer, 1981,

1984). He calls it a movement of retreat because, as experience is teaching us, the difficult, common search for insight into what is truly human and good is often broken off prematurely because everyone starts insisting on his or her rights. The question "who may decide?" thus short circuits the discussion what is "the good and humane to decide". The question then becomes one of competency, debating who has the right to decide, rather than a discussion that is concerned with the fundamental aspects of the matter. In a Christian view ethical analysis is more than a matter of procedural analysis. It is a question of what is the right thing to do. The exclusive affirmation of the autonomy principle can, indeed, prevent us from seeing the wonder of being human in its multi-sidedness. To grasp the whole of this mystery, we must consider as well the openness of each human being toward fellow-humans. As early as 1923, the Jewish philosopher, Martin Buber, wrote his pioneering work on being human, *I and Thou*, wherein he presented his relational philosophy. As humans, we essentially stand in an open relation, involved with the reality in which we live, with other humans to whom we owe our existence and who continue to surround us, and ultimately with God. If humans wish to be fully themselves, they stand in need of encounter with others and of being encountered by others. This is a fundamental insight that can guide us in our approach of the dying.

1. Care for the Dying as an Interhuman Event

Very often, the world of the dying person is wrongly assessed through the eyes of bystanders. The world of the dying person is frequently misunderstood. The following story is typical: the patient is a general practitioner in his final days. He is dying of cancer. He takes leave of the world in his diary in beautiful, frequently emotional terms. He describes how he is inevitably concerned with euthanasia, his own euthanasia: "Society has become aware of the ethical problems that confront doctors and patients. The overall approach to these problems is more nuanced than formerly. This is especially the case in regard to abortion and euthanasia. As a doctor I followed and acclaimed the growing liberalization in regard to these problems. But as a patient, to my surprise, I appear to be somewhat less "progressive": as a champion of free abortion for every woman who opts for it, in my family I would have felt the necessary difficulties, as a champion of euthanasia under strictly reglemented conditions, I clearly have difficulties in applying my criteria to myself". A

number of elements make clear how frequently and how easily people
speak about the dying, but how little the voice of the dying themselves is
heard. Or, how frequently people speak of the process of dying without
really being in the situation.

The world of the dying person is indeed frequently limited to his or her
bed and the few square meters that surround it. Everything that goes on in
this world – a big world for the dying person himself, even though it may
be considered unsightly and enormously limited in the eyes of the
bystanders – carries possibilities within itself, however small and
insignificant they may appear in the eyes of the nondying, that may reveal
the spacious and broad dimensions of meaningfulness, purification and
rest. Too often, the wrong criteria are used to judge the engagement of
those who sit by the deathbed for hours, those who can bring human
nearness alive with a small gesture. For the dying person, all of this has a
totally different dimension than what may simply be observed.

The exchange between the one seeming in need of help and the one
who is offering assistance, between the dying person and the accompanying person, is strongly influenced by the questions posed to the companion. The most difficult kinds of questions are obviously those which
touch the companion as a human being. This mainly occurs in borderline
situations, especially with regard to the meaning of life. The person who
has the courage to go into these questions does not escape the confrontation with the meaning of his or her own existence. Where the dying
person may becoming a question to him- or herself, this simultaneously
happens to the accompanying person as well. Being with a dying person,
therefore, really means actually participating in the event of dying: the
companion comes to deal with his or her own death, the paradox that
every human has to face.

Therefore, a humane accompaniment of the dying is not possible unless
the relationship between the dying person and the companion is taken
with utmost seriousness. To understand this, I refer again to the
anthropological model of the interwoveness of the three basic characteristics of our being human. The accompaniment of the dying is a very good
example of the relational character of our human condition of existence.
To clarify this point I shall first deal with the change that has come about
in the philosophical understanding of the term responsibility and then
apply it to caring for the dying as an expression of adoption of this
responsibility.

a. Responding to the Appeal of the Dying Person

Until recent times the physician attended to a patient on the basis of his
own specialty: he knew (and still knows) what is best for the patient on
the basis of his insight into what is good for his health. In other words, the
responsibility of the assistant was formulated in the first person "I (as
doctor, nurse ... member of the family) take the responsibility for such
and such a decision, for this unique person or this concrete action". The
patient entrusted himself fully to this strange world full of expertise
without, however, considering himself to be a partner in the process of
treatment. The Western, and essentially American, ethical reaction on this
situation was very hard and very strong: the principle of autonomy was
unfortunately used as an ethical instrument to change the medical
paternalism in a paternalism by the patient.

In my opinion this self-determination by the patient is indeed not a
fully adequate answer to medical paternalism. It is more an expression of
a one-sided anthropological insight in human existence than a good
pathway for the patient-physician relationship. This change can also be
described in the medical experience. Therefore, the concept of responsibility needs to be reconsidered in the line of relational philosophy. This
concept of responsibility underwent indeed fundamental alterations. The
new expression is no longer: "I am responsible", but "I have been made
responsible by the patient", (i.e., with all of my expertise I lend myself to
the promotion of the well-being of the patient). In this way the patient has
become a real and full partner in the counselling process and in the care
of his health.

Use is made here of a way of thinking already familiar in philosophical
thought, (i.e., the writings of M. Buber and E. Levinas). The ethical
relationship is interpreted as a relationship in which the other offers
himself to me in his being other. Thus he no longer subjects himself to a
meaning relative to my attitude to him. That most proper to the coun-
tenance of the other is that it appeals to me, hence ethical appeal: to what
extent do I permit myself to be appealed to by the patient who has
entrusted himself to my care? Through this appeal the patient directs
himself radically towards me. Thus I can perhaps run away from my
responsibility, but I can never pretend it does not exist.

One of the most essential conditions for the development of this
encounter is, thus, undoubtedly that the attendant knows himself made
responsible for the patient. This means that one attempts to respond to the

appeal that comes from the patient: that one turns to him with a willingness to meet him, to devote attention and care to him. It is the disinterested and affective reply to the need for real human closeness and assistance. An expert reply – and expertise in itself – thus remain a prerequisite. But the relative value of this expertise must be situated correctly: fundamentally one is dealing with an *interhuman* event involving both attendant and dying person. This relationship, furthermore, is entirely ethical in nature: the other confronts me and encounters me as a radical arrest of my egocentric desires, but he can do this only from a situation of extreme vulnerability. This insight requires clearly no explanation in the area of health-care.

Thus the intensity which the concept of ethical appeal can attain should be clear. In any case, health-care is placed in a new perspective – it is no longer the intention of the attendants or the maintenance of the institution that is primary, but rather the well-being of each patient and the promotion of more dignity.

b. When the Patient Beholds me

The companion will need courage to allow him or herself to face the questions raised by the demand for help from the dying person. Often, we all too easily flaunt the situation with words like "hope", "resurrection", "another life", while we pass by the doubtful and fearful questions on the human level. A closer analysis, therefore, explains why I prefer to describe this as an interhuman event, in which both the one who asks for help as well as the companion are fully implicated. Dialogues between the patient and those who accompany him function as a form in which the personal encounter between two humans becomes flesh and blood and receives its concrete shape.

It is at the same time the background against which I would like to situate therapeutic obstinacy and would like to formulate an ethical stand for the companionship with the dying person. It is also the fundamental background against which I will consider the specific dilemmas in the shortening of the dying process.

2. Situating Therapeutic Obstinacy

As in every emotionally loaded problem, the risk of one-sidedness is not just imaginary. One-sidedness can have many causes: it can come from an insufficiently founded insight into the problem, from one's own philosophy of life and/or an ethical point of view which views life as an absolute value, or from a predisposition which hangs together with one's own attitude toward life, illness, or death (Sporken, 1981).

Thus, for example, the problem of euthanasia is falsely put if it is suggested that dying people must make a choice between dying in unbearable pain or actively shortening the dying process. This is an argument that is often encountered among the ranks of those who propagate the social acceptance of a voluntary "easy death". The real answer to heavy and unbearable bodily suffering lies, in the Christian tradition, not in the social acceptance of euthanasia but in professional and carefully applied palliative care. Relatively few physicians are skilled in the use of narcotics or pain killing drugs. This has grown to be an area of research in itself, and it is here that an important alternative can be found (see O'Rourke, this volume). This also applies to the psycho-social suffering of a dying person: it is first and foremost an appeal to those who accompany the dying person for human proximity and companionship. To answer this appeal by offering voluntary euthanasia is an escape from the real question and a sign of impotence with regard to the humane accompaniment of the patient. Such a suggestion does not solve the lacunae in medical training or the incapacity to deal with the dying person.

Another false question is set up by those who counter the suggestion of (active or passive) euthanasia with a determined effort to use every medical tool for keeping a patient alive, even when it is clear that death is inevitable. This mentality is often inspired by absolutizing the norm of "respect for life" (the sanctity of life-principle) and subsequently leaves very little room for accepting the process of dying in a manner that is humanly worthy.

Finally, it is equally one-sided to oppose the autonomy of the patient over against what is usually called medical power. Here, the right to self-determination is formulated in such a radical way that it seems as if every human being would be living on an island. Therefore again, I would give more attention to the dying as an interhuman event: humans are relational beings, they need others in order to reach the fulfillment of life. The affirmation of a radicalized notion of freedom – legally translated into the right of self-determination – detracts from this and leads to a profound impoverishment of the mystery that humans represent in all their relations and dimensions.

3. Shortening the Dying Process: An Ethical Perspective

The decision on the ethical justifiability of using all possible means to prolong life involves not simply an evaluation of the physical existence but that of the whole person. Therefore, it is good to be aware of an entire complex of values and norms with regard to life. Biological life implies a call to humanization. Our relational-personalistic approach has now to be translated in an ethical guideline for dealing with the problem of excessive medical technology.

First, at a given moment, a situation may arise in which it may be possible to prolong life or the dying process for a shorter or longer period of time by applying medical means or by fighting possible complications. Usually, the ethical question is formulated as follows: on the basis of what arguments is it ethically justifiable to refrain from employing life-sustaining measures? This question follows from a certain ethical vision that physicians are bound to do whatever they can. This opinion was reasonable at a time when there were relatively few techniques available for postponing an inevitable death for a certain period of time. Today, however, the possibilities for prolonging biological life have expanded tremendously. It therefore appears necessary to reformulate the ethical question and to ask: on what grounds should a physician artificially prolong an inevitably terminal process? This question presupposes a different ethical background, namely, the understanding that one is only obliged to use the available medical means for the prolongation of life if the well-being of the patient (individually or socially) is genuinely being served. The point of departure here is the respect for the person and the process of dying as interhuman event (Verspieren, 1984, 1985).

A second observation would be that, when a decision must be made about a treatment, the doctor has to weigh the various values and disvalues which are at stake – including all the important elements: personal and familial as well as medical and that he/she must consider the extent to which a particular treatment might promote human fulfillment. This proportionate judgment needs to be made in each particular case: one will evaluate the possibilities by considering the type of treatments available, their degree of complexity, the costs, and their possibilities of application along with the result that can be expected, taking into account the condition of the sick person and his or her bodily and moral strength (Sacred Congregation for the Doctrine of the Faith, 1980). The attending physician, therefore, will need to consider to what degree any treatment can still be meaningful, guided by a deep respect for facilitating a process of dying that is worthy of human beings. Obviously, one cannot do this alone. The collaboration with colleagues, nurses, patients and family is essential, which is another symbol of responsible involvement.These are the two fundamental steps in the ethical decision making: Assessing whether or not one should sustain life and assessing biological life in view of other values. Then comes the third step: making the decision. It seems a good suggestion to reconsider this process 48 hours after this decision. The responsibility for this decision lies in my view in the hands of the physician. He/she is indeed the only one in the situation who has the skill, the experience and the responsibility to bear the load of such decisions. Some people would call this an example of medical paternalism. I don't think it is right to react in that way. Parents of dying children are not prepared to make such decisions and to be confronted with this cruel dilemmas. Children of dying patients sometime also avoid this kind of involvement. Of course, it has been made clear enough that the structure of this decision is fully relational. The exercise of medicine in such cases, is in my view, indeed, fully relational: as a caring and curing profession medicine is a symbol of the relational structure of the human person, as I have described this.

I will now apply the three-step structure of these kinds of decisions in the context of dying as an interhuman event on the problem of the PVS patient and his nutrition or hydration.

4. Ethical Dilemmas at the Edges of Life: The PVS Patient and the Nutrition/Hydration Debate

With the development of the technology of life-support during the last 30 years, severely ill persons have survived in coma, in the chronic vegetative state, or in other states of great impairment. These persons formerly would have died relatively promptly after the insult that precipitated their condition. Now they are shielded from cardiopulmonary collapse and death by modern forms of life support, which extend from complex volume ventilators to simple methods of feeding by gastrostomy tube (Carton, 1990; see also, Storey, this volume). Today, 85% to 90% of critical care professionals state that they are withholding and withdrawing life sustaining treatment from patients who are deemed to have irreversible disease and are terminally ill. Thus, during the past 15 years we have evolved from situations in which it was a deviation from the medical and ethical standard to withdraw a respirator, nutrition, or intravenous fluids from a nonbrain dead patient to the present environment, in which it is accepted practice and becoming the norm to withdraw such medical treatments in certain groups of patients (Sprung, 1990). In a recent study, Smedira and others concluded that although life-sustaining care is withheld or withdrawn relatively infrequently from patients in the intensive care unit, such decisions precipitate about half of all deaths in the intensive care units of the hospitals they studied. In most of these cases the patients were incompetent, but physicians and families usually agreed to limit care (Smedira, 1990).

A first and important ambiguity about PVS patients is if they can be considered as dying patients. This is extremely important. Depending on the answer on this question, this dilemma becomes very easy to react upon; it would be only one of the several possible applications of our ethical perspective (the promotion of a humane dying process). Indeed, we can apply then our ethical perspective and describe nutrition and hydration for the PVS patients in terms of proportionality and proportionate reason.

The difference between a dying and non-dying patient roots in a value judgment about whether we ought to use the available technology or not. The category "the dying patient" can not be presented as if it were independently of value judgments and descriptively clear (McCormick, 1989). Concerning the PVS patient the ambiguity is, however, enormous. Shannon and Walter suggest clearly that they believe that the PVS patient is not dying: "An important fact about a PVS patient is that he or she is not dying. In these patients the brain stem is intact, with the major damage to the brain occurring in the neocortex and cortex. Thus these patients breath spontaneously, have their eyes open, have a sleep-wake cycle, their pupils respond to light, and they typically have a normal gag and cough reflex" (Shannon and Walter, 1988).

It is further of critical importance to know whether these patients experience pain and/or suffering. Cranford, following the amicus curiae brief of the American Academy of Neurology in the Paul Brophy Case, argues that PVS patients "may" "react" to painful and other noxious stimuli, but they do not "feel" (experience) pain in the sense of conscious discomfort ..., because the centers of the brain required for these experiences are too compromised to be functional (Cranford, 1988).

It is, however, not uncommon for PVS patients to survive in their vegetative condition for five, ten, and twenty years. With Shannon and

Walter we can resume the ethical dilemma as such: "... we obviously have the medical capacity to provide nutrition and hydration for these individuals, but the ethical difficulty, of course, is whether we must do everything we can to sustain their existence in this clinical condition" (see also, Bole, Paris, Wildes, this volume).

I would essentially stress the fact that an external intervention is needed to prevent the PVS patient from dying. It is almost impossible to restore meaningful life for the PVS patient. In any case, following our first guideline (on what grounds should a physician artificially prolong an inevitably terminal process?), it would be better to make clear this before the decision is made to introduce a feeding tube. The fundamental value question remains indeed: on what grounds should a physician artificially prolong an inevitable terminal process? The decision (not) to introduce the feeding tube, to withhold or withdraw treatment, has to be made after weighing values and disvalues. The focus of the decision should, however, be *the humane dying process*. Instead of using artificial feeding to show caring, plans can be made for supportive care – pain control, skin care, and personal hygiene. Even when artificial feeding is not used to treat malnutrition and dehydratation, the symptoms of hunger and thirst can be relieved by moistening the patient's mouth with ice chips or, when possible, with oral food and fluids. It is good to remember here the unconscious mechanisms that can play through this kind of decisions, as Schneiderman made clear: "I submit that in deliberately prescribing treatments that prolong the lives of patients in a vegetative state, we are causing the persistent vegetative state; thus we are unwittingly yet cruelly resurrecting the archaic practice of banishment" (Schneiderman, 1990).

The relational approach of the dying in general and of the PVS patient in particular confronts us with the central question if there is still a possibility to develop a relational encounter with the patient. The PVS patient has lost his personality, became totally dependant, cannot organize his own life. He is no longer a free human being. He has even lost the possibility to feed himself. He is socially dead and lives only further at the frontiers of a biological death. He is not suffering. Care for the dying as an interhuman event is no longer possible. The fact that free will, relational potentiality and communication are totally absent, creates a totally new situation. Real care for these patients could be made possible through the acceptance that this is a radical new situation. Family and others in his neighborhood have to start the process of mourning in the face of a person who is still biologically alive. Nutrition and hydration are the symbolic relational exchanges from the external world to keep this human being biologically alive. The new identity of the PVS patient makes it, however, impossible to establish a really interhuman relationship. The acceptance that the human person has died, but the biological identity is still present, must make possible to accept that care has only become a means of external intervention without which the PVS patient would not survive biologically. To put this in the terms of the Vatican Declaration on Euthanasia: "in any case, it will be possible to make a correct judgment as to the means by studying the type of treatment to be used, its degree of complexity or risk, its cost and the possibilities of using it, and comparing these elements with the result that can be expected, taking into account the state of the sick person and his or her physical and moral resources" (Sacred Congregation for the Doctrine of the Faith, 1980). This makes clear that, when no relational structure is possible any more, there is no longer the duty to prolong biological life.

CONCLUSION

A humane accompaniment of the dying is not possible unless the relationship between the dying person and his bystanders is taken with utmost seriousness. The work required will take a great deal of effort on the part of all involved. I wanted to present my approach as a realistic alternative for the progress of the radical idea of autonomy and self-determination, which leads to the acceptance of active euthanasia. Dying is indeed only human when it is lived trough as an interhuman event.

It can be true to say that the debate on nutrition and hydration for the PVS patient confronts us with a difficult dilemma. The real challenge for our society is, however, the promotion of humanity in dying. This is the crucial task for the future. Every human being is a promise that cannot be kept ... this becomes clear when one of our beloved is dying and it will even be more clear, when we are dying ourselves. Divine Grace can be experienced by recognizing my own responsibility for the well-being of the other who sometimes beholds me as a dying human being.

BIBLIOGRAPHY

Apostel, L., Devroey, P. and Cammaer, H. (eds.): 1987, *Beschikken over lijf en leven. Ethische vragen rond vrijheid en geborgenheid*, Acco, Leuven.
Aries, Ph.: 1977, *L'homme devant la mort*, Paris.

Aries, Ph.: 1983, *Imaqes de l'homme devant la mort*, Paris.

Beauchamp, T. L. and Childress J. F.: 1983, *Principles of Biomedical Ethics*, Oxford University Press, New York.

Boné, E.: 1989, *Dignity and Solidarity at the Edges of Life, Symposion Report*, Ad Instar Manuscripti, Brussels.

Bopp, J.: 1990, 'Choosing death for Nancy Cruzan', *Hastings Center Report* 20, nr.1, 42–44.

Callahan, D.: 1983, 'On feeding the dying', *Hastings Center Report* 13, 22.

Connery, J. R.: 1980, 'Prolonging life: The duty of its limits', *Linacre Quarterly*, 47, 151–165.

Connery, J. R.: 1983, 'The teleology of proportionate reason', *Theological Studies* 44, 489–496.

Connery, J. R.: 1986 'Quality of life', *Linacre Quarterly* 53, 31–36.

Demeester-De Meyer, W. (ed.): 1987, *Bioethica in de Jaren '90. 2 Vols.*, Omega Editions, Gent.

De Wachter, M. A. M.: 1989, 'Active euthanasia in the Netherlands', *The Journal of the American Medical Association* 262(23), 3316–3319.

Diekstra, R. (ed.): 1983, *De zelfgekozen dood. De problematiek en de hulpverlening*, Ambo, Baarn.

Eijk, W. J.: 1987, *De zelfgekozen dood naar aanleiding van een dodelijke en ongeneeslijke ziekte. Een medisch-historisch en medisch-ethisch onderzoek ten behoeve van een Rooms-Katholiek standpunt inzake euthanasie*, Tabor, Brugge.

Fenigsen, R.: 1987, *Euthanasie: een weldaad?*, Van Loghum Slaterus, Deventer.

Fenigsen, R.: 1989, 'A Case Against Dutch Euthanasia', *Hastings Center Report, A Special Supplement* 19, 22–30.

'Final Report of the Netherlands State Commission on Euthanasia. An English Summary', *Bioethics* 1, 162–174.

Gevers, J. K. M.: 1987, 'Legal developments concerning active euthanasia on request in the Netherlands', *Bioethics* 1, 156–162.

Ghoos, J.: 1986, *In de schaduw van de dood*, Davidsfonds, Leuven.

Häring, B.: 1973, *Medical Ethics*, Fides, Notre Dame.

Jennett, B. & Plum, F.: 1972, 'Persistent vegetative state after brain damage. A syndrome in search of a name', *Lancet*, 480–484.

Kuhse, H.: 1987, *The Sanctity-of-Life Doctrine in Medicine. A Critique*, Clarendon Press, Oxford.

Kuhse, H. & Singer, P.: 1990, 'Editorial', *Bioethics*, 4, nr. 3, III.

Kuitert, H. M.: 1981, *Een gewenste dood. Euthanasie en zelfbeschikking als moreel en godsdienstig probleem*, Ambo, Baarn.

McCormick, R. A.: 1975, 'A proposal for "Quality of Life" criteria for sustaining life', *Hospital Progress* 56, 76–79.

Paris, J. J. and Mc Cormick, R. A.: 1987, 'The Catholic tradition on the use of nutrition and fluids', *America* 156, 356–361.

Ramsey, P.: 1978, *Ethics at the Edges of Life: Medical and Legal Intersections*, New Haven, 181–187.

Rapport van de Nederlandse Staatscommissie Euthanasie, 's Gravenhage, 1985.

Rigter, H.: 1989, 'Euthanasia in the Netherlands', *Hastings Center Report. A Special Supplement* 19, 31–32.

Rolies, J. and Pijnenburg, M: 1985, 'Euthanasie-rapport van de Nederlandse staatscommissie', *Kultuurleven* 52, 847–857.

Shannon, T. A. and Walter, J. J.: 1988, 'The PVS patient and the forgoing/withdrawing of medical nutrition and hydration', *Theological Studies* 49, 623–647.

Steinbrook, R. and Lo, B.: 1988, 'Artificial feeding-solid ground, not a slippery slope', *The New England Journal of Medicine* 318, 286–290.

Van Der Wal, G. A. *et al.* (eds.): 1987, *Euthanasie. Knelpunten in een discussie*, Ambo, Baarn.

Veatch, R. M.: 1989, Death, *Dying and the Bioloaical Revolution. Our Last Quest for Responsibility*, Yale University Press, New York.

Verspieren, P.: 1984, *Face à celui qui meurt. Euthanasie, Acharnement Thérapeutique, Accompagnement*, Desdeé De Brouwer, Paris.

Verspieren, P.: 1985, 'Euthanasie. Le délot éthique', *Etudes* 362, 479–492.

KEVIN Wm. WILDES S.J.

LIFE AS A GOOD AND OUR OBLIGATIONS TO PERSISTENTLY VEGETATIVE PATIENTS

INTRODUCTION

With the development of medical technology it is possible to maintain the life of a patient in a persistent vegetative state for an indefinite period of time. A persistent vegetative state (PVS) is a one of permanent unconsciousness with a loss of all cerebral cortical functions, which leads to complete unawareness of self or of the environment, though there is the persistence of sleep-wake cycles (Executive Board, American Academy of Neurology, 1989, pp. 125–126). There are 15,000–25,000 PVS patients in the United States (AMA Council on Scientific Affairs and Council on Ethical and Judicial Affairs, p. 427). As the recent discussions about the case of Nancy Cruzan illustrate, such cases raise difficult moral and legal questions for the families of such patients as well as for medical and legal communities and society at large (Cruzan). The ethical, political, and judicial arguments over these cases have raised discussion about the extent of our obligation to treat such patients.

Discussions of the nature and extent of treatment obligations towards persistently vegetative patients have engendered a body of literature which argues that human life is a basic good, intrinsic to the person (e.g. May *et al.*, 1987; Grisez, 1989; McHugh, 1989). Those who hold this position argue that life should be understood as a basic human good which cannot be acted against directly; that is, the prohibition against taking life is absolute. On this view the withdrawal or withholding of medically assisted nutrition and hydration is an act of killing by omission and since human life is a good of the person remaining alive such a life should never be regarded as a burden (May *et al.*, pp. 204–205). The conclusion then drawn is that there is an obligation to sustain the life of PVS patients by means of artificial nutrition and hydration.

There are many controversial points to this position. For example, there are questions about conclusions drawn from these arguments that omissions of artificial nutrition and hydration for PVS patients are acts of "killing" which cannot be described under the distinction of ordinary-

K.Wm. Wildes (ed.), Birth, Suffering and Death, 145–154.

extraordinary means (Grisez, 1989, p. 174; see T. Bole; this volume; J. Paris, this volume). There are also questions about the "burdensome" nature of artificial feeding and hydration (see, P. Storey, this volume) and how such patients are understood within the Catholic tradition (see, J. Paris, this volume). The focus of this essay, however, is not upon these questions. Rather it is to examine the fundamental claim that biological human life, that is, life *simpliciter* sans any sentience or potential for sentience, should be understood as a basic human good. In such a view human biological life is understood as a sufficient reason, by itself, for determining action.

To justify for this position, those who hold it argue first that there are "basic human goods". They distinguish the "basic" human goods from all other goods (objects of interest) in two ways. First the basic human goods are integral for fulfillment (Finnis *et al.*, pp. 277–278, 305). Second these goods are principles of practical reason; that is, they provide a reason for action which requires no other. The first principle of common morality, as formulated by Finnis, Boyle, Grisez, is: "In acting for human goods and avoiding what is opposed to them, *one ought to choose and otherwise will those and only those possibilities whose willing is compatible with integral human fulfillment*" (p. 283). The basic human goods give content to the concept of integral human fulfillment though the authors are clear to say that fulfillment is not an additive sum of the basic human goods. The authors set out a list of what they consider to be basic human goods: truth, friendship, life, knowledge, excellence in performance, peace, and fraternity (Finnis *et al.*, pp. 279–280). From this list the authors believe one can deduce principles and rules governing human actions. The principle with which we are concerned is the prohibition against taking innocent human life.

There are important philosophical questions about the authors' arguments and conclusions about the content of practical reason. In a post-modern age, one can ask if there is a "common morality". In such a morally pluralistic age, how is it possible to speak, in any shared and content-full way, about integral human fulfillment and human nature? It turns out that any normative account of human nature already presupposes a normative interpretation of that nature. That is, one must already stand within a particular moral framework in order to understand how normatively to assess human nature and its moral implications. Within a particular moral viewpoint (e.g., the Christian moral viewpoint) there may be a reflective equilibrium between human nature morally understood and other moral intuitions and principles, such that a full and coherent account can be elaborated. In a purely secular, pluralistic context, one finds numerous competing interpretations of human nature and basic human goods. One cannot choose among them without having already taken a particular moral stand. Finnis, Boyle, and Grisez need to acknowledge the extent to which their arguments are embedded within a particular moral tradition and its richness. Even apart from this general theoretical observation, however, the arguments of Finnis *et al.* suffer from significant difficulties which should be explored.

The defining condition for a human good as "basic" is that it be both a principle of practical reason *and* an element of integral human fulfillment. "As a principle of practical reasoning, a basic human good can provide for choices a reason requiring no further reasons" (Finnis *et al.*, p. 304). As an element of integral fulfillment "its instantiations are intrinsic to persons and fulfill an essential aspect of human nature" (Finnis *et al.*, p. 304). One difficulty in following the argument is that the authors shift back and forth between the two criteria.

Does human biological life meet these two criteria? What does it mean that life is a principle of practical reason? When someone rescues a person from a life threatening situation the rescuer may say that she preformed her heroics in order to save the life of the other. But does the rescuer mean to save biological life alone or the whole matrix of human goods and fulfillment which constitutes the life of the person rescued? We assume something like the latter sense of life and not the former. One can conceive of having and desiring the other basic goods for their own sake. One can conceive, for example, of friendship or truth abstractly pursued *in se*; that is, as a sufficient reason for action. But do we understand human biological life by itself, stripped of all of the goods to which it can lead, as something to be pursued for its own sake? I do not think our heroic rescuer risked his own life for "life" on the biological level *simpliciter*. It is not obvious that one should risk one's *own life* for another's life it the other were capable of nothing else but life.

The authors hold that as a principle of practical reason, "one need not look to any other good to find a reason ..." (Finnis *et al.*, p. 305). It seems clear, however, that life does not meet this criteria in the way other goods are principles of practical reason for we act to save life not for itself but as a basis of other goods. Finnis *et al.* respond to this criticism by saying that one should not demand too much from any one basic good; that is, no single good captures all the richness and rational ground provided by "integral human fulfillment" (Finnis, p. 305). This response, however, does not answer the objection since this response shifts from the criterion of practical reason to the criterion of integral fulfillment. It has not been claimed that, considered in abstraction, any of the basic goods yields the fullness of integral human fulfillment. Rather, the objection claims that the other basic goods give some reason for acting, by themselves, which human biological life, by itself, does not give. People desire not only to live but to live well and in so doing to achieve spiritual ends. It does seem that in considering life in abstraction we do think of it as a *necessary*, but not sufficient, condition for action.

The authors give a second and more detailed argument for why they consider life as a basic human good through a *reductio as absurdum* argument. The authors set out two ways of conceiving life; that is, as a basic human good and as an instrumental good (p. 307 ff.). They argue that to hold the position that human life is an instrumental good leads to a rationally indefensible conception of human beings as dualistic beings in which "person" is distinct from "life". Their argument seems to be as follows:

1. Assume that life is best understood as an instrumental good.
2. Life is a human good which has to do with the well-being of the person.
3. On the instrumental view the "life" of the person must be extrinsic to the person.
4. This (#3) commits us to a dualism of person and life since on the instrumentalist account life is extrinsic to the person.
5. Such dualism is incoherent since human beings are not two realities.
6. Life must be conceived as a basic human good.

Now there is a significant assumption made in this argument. In their characterization the authors clearly set up a notion of "instrumental" as being extrinsic to the person (pp. 307–308). Earlier in the text they conceive instrumentality in terms of "possessions" and "things". With this literal characterization of instrumentalism the dualism they find indefensible becomes inevitable. The absurdity they demonstrate rests on the assumption that the dualism of life and person is necessarily ontological. But why must this be the case? Could there not be a conceptual distinction of the two without having a commitment to an ontological dualism? There is a significant difference between drawing a conceptual distinction and holding that the conceptual distinction has ontological status; that is, that the distinction implies the existence of two substances. One can distinguish many different roles within the life of most adults (e.g., husband, parent, physician, friend, neighbor), however, we do not think that for each conceptual distinction a separate "reality" exists. The strength of their argument relies on the ontological implication. They have, however, given no reason to draw such strong ontological conclusions.

HUMAN LIFE: A CATEGORIAL UNDERSTANDING

The difficulty with affirming that life is a good lies in trying to give an account of the type of "good" which it is. According to the criteria established by Finnis, Boyle and Grisez, human biological life does not seem to be a basic human good because it does not, by itself, provide a practical reason for action. Nor does life seem to be a good which is merely an object of interest. Many people have objects of interest towards which we have no obligation to help them realize (Nagel, 1988). Yet, we hold that we do have obligations to help others protect and preserve their lives. It seems that "life" as a good falls somewhere between an object of interest and a basic human good. An alternative approach to explaining biological life as a good is captured through understanding human life categorially.

The mind can only know through concepts. A categorial explanation seeks to interpret a situation by the relation of foundational concepts; that is, to integrate different levels of meaning and concepts. A categorial account seeks to give a conceptual reconstruction propose a conceptual model of reality. Human biological life is one category of our experience. By itself it is an incomplete reconstruction of human life for mere biological life is a moment, a condition, of human life fully realized and understood. Human personal life is the higher truth of human biological life but human biological life *simpliciter* is not human personal life. Nor is human biological life a thing over against and distinct from human personal life. Instead, human personal life is a categorial fulfillment of human biological life. The two contrast as dialectically bound categories of reality. The first fulfilling and presupposing the other; the other, incomplete without the first. One does not have a dualism of things but a relationship between distinct categories. By invoking the language of ontological dualism, one reifies intertwined levels of reality and in doing so structurally obscures the matters at issue.

In the ordinary routine of life the integration of these factors (life,

goods, well being) is such that the life of a person encompasses all of
them in an integrated fashion in a way that does not draw attention to
their distinctiveness. It is in sickness that we can experience the distinctions. For example when the goals and projects one pursues are put to the
side because of the effects of illness one experiences one's body as an
instrument which fails to support the realization of one's goals. In
extreme moments of bodily dysfunction the pursuit of any good may
become impossible (e.g., p.v.s. patients). We can begin to see, in reflecting on illness, why one may speak of life as a necessary, through not
sufficient, condition for the pursuit of any good and the possibility of
integral human fulfillment. Biological life is an "instrument" for attaining
such goods and their fulfillment. A categorial reconstruction of human
life would hold that human biological life is a good because it is a
necessary condition for all other goods of human life. As such, human
biological life deserves protection and support in a way that other goods
(objects of interest) do not. Without biological life none of the other
goods are attainable. Simultaneously, human life is incomplete when the
category of personal life is no longer possible. Thus, we are not obliged to
treat human biological life as a good which trumps all others and should
be maintained for its own sake.

Undoubtedly this position will be cast as instrumentalist; however, one
must be careful how that term is understood. Finnis, Boyle and Grisez
build in to instrumentalism certain ontological assumptions that need not
be accepted. In a classic formulation, John Dewey put forth a theory of
instrumentalism precisely to overcome dualistic thinking (Dewey, 1960,
pp. 195–223). Instrumentalism is, rather, a condition of reasoning. In the
Deweyian formulation theories, ideas, and concepts are *analogous* to
tools and instruments. Dewey certainly did not conceive them as extrinsic
to a person as Finnis, Boyle and Grisez, interpret the term (Finnis *et al.* p.
304). We can distinguish at least three dimensions of human life: the
biological life of a human being, one's integral human fulfillment, and the
pursuit of goods as conditions of that fulfillment. Conceptually distinguishing these dimensions, however, does not imply that they are
ontologically distinct as Finnis *et al.* assume. Rather, the categorical
distinctions allow us to reconstruct the mystery of human life.

If one conceives of biological life as an instrumental good one can still
maintain a distinction of basic human goods and goods as objects of
interest. The basic human goods, (e.g., friendship, truth), are practical
reasons for acting and essential to human fulfillment. Life becomes a

necessary, underlying condition for these goods and human fulfillment. Does this understanding of life threaten the need to safeguard and protect human life? No. As the authors themselves admit, to take innocent human life is to act against a necessary condition for all human goods, basic and otherwise. The conceptualization of biological life as a necessary condition of human, personal life generates a strong argument to protect such life without generating a perfect obligation to sustain life.

THE PVS PATIENT

In what way does a categorial understanding of human biological life and human personal life affect how we conceive our obligations to those patients who are in persistent vegetative states? In a later article, specifically addressing the care PVS patient, G. Grisez (1989) sets out to clarify the philosophical issues underlying the collective statement (May et al., 1987). Much of what he says involves a restatement of the earlier criticisms of the dualism and instrumentality.

There are, however, some important new elements in this later piece. Grisez does allow the possibility of a person removing medically assisted feeding and hydration, by means of a clear advanced directive. In this way a person may relieve the obligation of others to care for the patient should he come to be in a permanently vegetative state (p. 169). However, it seems clear then that his position is that life is a basic human good which we have an obligation to maintain and against which one may not act directly. Furthermore, he describes the removal of artificial feeding and hydration as an act of "killing". The language used in the description is crucial since the same actions can be described as a withdrawal of medical intervention (McCormick, 1985). The language that is used by Finnis, Boyle and Grisez is chosen so as to offset any argument about double effect, intentionality, and ordinary-extraordinary means distinction[1], (See J. Paris, T. Bole, this volume). What is curious about the language used by Grisez is that if the stopping of artificial feeding and hydration is "killing" why would he not consider the medical directive, of which he approves, which waives such treatment, as "suicide"? On a conceptual level it is not clear why Grisez should allow patients to make such decisions about their own treatment and not allow others to make the same judgment.

Grisez expresses other important concerns about how the ways we view life and the PVS patient will affect the way in which we view and treat the mentally disabled. He argues for a bond of "human solidarity" which would lead us to protect both types of patients. A crucial question, however, is whether or not society should view these two types of patients in the same way. There seems to be a significant distinction between them in that the PVS patient was, at one time, potentially capable of the basic human goods, other goods, or human fulfillment at some level. Now, however, because of fatal pathological conditions such patients are no longer capable of such goods or fulfillment at any level[2]. Because of the primary pathology the category of personal life, which is the higher truth and fulfillment of human biological life, is no longer possible for PVS patients. This in itself constitutes a pathology. May's concern for the slippery slope from the PVS patient to the mentally disabled is ill founded in that those who are mentally disabled are unlike PVS patients who lack any awareness of self, environment, or sensory stimuli (American Academy of Neurology, 1989). There is a second fatal pathology for PVS patients because the individuals who are so afflicted are not capable of life without some type of medical intervention (i.e. medically assisted feeding and hydration). The presence of this additional pathological condition further helps to distinguish PVS patients from those who are mentally disabled. Kevin O'Rourke summarizes this additional pathology when he writes: "If a fatal pathology is not present, whether in the person who is mentally competent or in the person who is mentally disabled, then nutrition and hydration should be provided by others if one cannot provide these goods of life for oneself" (O'Rourke, p. 182). A mentally disabled person may reach the PVS level or be materially equivalent to a PVS patient. In those cases, the categorical understanding of human life would argue that there is no obligation to sustain the life of such a patient by medical means.

In the tradition language of the Church, the soul is a principle of being because it is the principle of human life. Soul and body constitute a substantial unity in which the body is, as ensouled, the expression of a person's spiritual personality. The spiritual principle of the human being acts in space and time and seeks to brings the material, spatio-temporal being to perfection of the whole person. As a spiritual being the human person is open to the transcendence of God with freedom and responsibility. It seems crucial to remember that the brain is the integrating organ for the human being. It is the proper matter of the faculty of the rational soul. When it is medically clear that such matter has been destroyed, then it seems impossible to argue that a substantial union of body and soul remains or that an obligation to sustain life remains (B. Ashley, this volume).

CONCLUSION

There are those who have argued that there is an obligation to feed and hydrate PVS patients because life is a basic human good and they have advanced two arguments to support their position. First there is the argument that biological life is a principle of practical reason. However, it is not clear that mere biological life can be a principle of practical reason since it is a necessary reason and not a sufficient reason for choice. The second argument has held that life is a basic good because an "instrumentalist" account leads to a dualism. This argument, however, rests on a definition of instrumentalism which assumes an ontological dualism that need not be made. This argument faces the difficulty that it *assumes* that the dualism of person and biological life must have an ontological, not a conceptual, character.

As an alternative it has been proposed that the personal and biological categories be viewed as conceptually distinct. Human biological life is a necessary condition for the achievement of the basic human goods as well as integral human fulfillment. This position captures the complexities found in the experience of illness. It allows a more nuanced approach to separating the class of PVS patients from the mentally disabled and other vulnerable patients. It does not commit us to the perfect obligation of sustaining the life of the PVS patients.

NOTES

[1] In a classic article on this issue Gerald Kelly referred to such states as "terminal coma" (Kelly, 1950, p. 220). He argued that even if one considered medical treatments such as artificial hydration and feeding to be ordinary, they may, in certain circumstances be described as "a *useless* ordinary means" (Kelly, p. 219).

[2] By "fatal pathology" I understand any illness, disease, or lesion which will cause death unless it is removed or circumvented. The fatal pathology affecting the PVS patient is an inability to chew or swallow. These are purposeful human activities which are no longer possible if the cerebral cortex is unable to function (O'Rourke, p. 182).

BIBLIOGRAPHY

AMA, Council on Scientific Affairs and Council on Ethical and Judicial Affairs: 1990, 'Persistent vegetative state and the decision to withdraw or withhold life support', *The Journal of the American Medical Association*, Vol. 263, no. 3, January 19, 1990, 426–430.

Archdiocese of New York: 1990, 'Principles in regard to withholding or withdrawing artificially assisted nutrition/hydration', *Issues in Law and Medicine*, Vol 6, no. 1, 89–93.

Ashley, B.: 1991, 'Dominion or stewardship: Theological reflections', this volume, pp. 171–187.

Bole, T.: 1991, Why almost any cost to others to preserve the life of the irreversibly comatose constitutes an extraordinary means, this volume, pp.

Boyle, L.: 1989, 'Sanctity of Life and Suicide: Tensions and developments within common morality' in B.A. Brody (ed.), *Suicide and Euthanasia*, Kluwer Academic Publishers, Dordrecht, The Netherlands, pp. 221–250.

Dewey, J.: 1960, *The Quest for Certainty*, Putnamn, New York.

Engelhardt, H. T. 1973, *Mind-Body: A Categorial Relations*, Martinus Nijhoff, The Hague.

Executive Board, American Academy of Neurology.: 1989, 'Position statement on the management and care of persistent vegetative state patient', Neurology, 39, 125–126.

Finnis, J., J. Boyle, G. Grisez: 1987, *Nuclear Deterrence, Morality and Realism*, Clarendon Press, Oxford.

Grisez, G.: 1989, 'Should nutrition and hydration be provided to the permanently unconscious and other mentally disabled persons? ', *Issues in Law and Medicine*, 5, 165–179.

Kelly, G.: 1950, 'The duty of using artificial means of preserving life', *Theological Studies*, 11, 203–220.

May, W. *et al.*: 1987, 'Feeding and hydrating the permanently unconscious and other vulnerable persons', *Issues in Law and Medicine*, 3, 204–2 17.

May, W.: 1990, 'Criteria for withholding or withdrawing treatment', *Linacre Quarterly*, Vol. 57, No. 3, 81–90.

McCormick, R.: 1985, 'Caring or starving? The case of Claire Conroy', *America*, April 6, 269–273.

McHugh, J. T.: 1989, 'Artificially assisted nutrition and hydration', *Origins*, 19, 213–216.

Nancy Beth Cruzan v. Director Missouri Department of Health: 1990, 58 Law Week, June 25, 1990, 4916–4941.

Nagel, T.: 1988, 'Autonomy and deontology', *Consequentialism and Its Critics*, S. Scheffler (ed), Oxford University Press, New York, pp. 142–172.

O'Rourke, K.: 1989, 'Should nutrition and hydration be provided to permanently unconscious and other mentally disabled persons?', *Issues in Law and Medicine*, 5, 181–196.

Paris, J.: 1991, 'The catholic tradition on the use of nutrition and fluids', this volume pp. 189–208.

Storey, P.: 1991, 'Artificial feeding and hydration in advanced illness', this volume pp. 67–75.

SECTION III

MORAL QUANDARIES

KEVIN D. O'ROURKE O.P.

PAIN RELIEF: ETHICAL ISSUES AND CATHOLIC TEACHING

INTRODUCTION

When caring for a sick person, a physician seeks to cure the person by eliminating or alleviating the illness, disease or injury which causes dysfunction on the part of the patient. But the physician also assumes the responsibility to alleviate the pain which results from the original disease or injury, or from the therapy which is directed toward cure. For several centuries, physicians were more able to assuage pain than they were to remove or alleviate the source of it. In the latter half of this century remarkable progress has been made in alleviating and removing pain. Determining which medications to use, to relieve serious pain, and how much to use, is now a subspecialty in contemporary medicine (Bonica, 1990; Loeser, 1989). The use of medication to relieve pain however, gives rise to two ethical issues: 1) pain medication may impair a patient's cognitive function, thus making it difficult for the person to prepare for death; 2) pain medication may hasten death. This presentation will study the two ethical issues in light of the teaching of the Catholic Church and explain the reasoning underlying this teaching.

I. THE ISSUES

Pain is anything that causes distress or suffering. Pain may occur in many different levels of human function. For example, people experience spiritual pain as they contemplate the guilt they have incurred through sin of the past, even though these sins have been forgiven. Again, people may experience emotional pain from the death of a friend or family member even though they realize, that given the person's debilitated condition, the person's death was a blessed and welcome event. In this essay, the subject of consideration is neither spiritual nor emotional pain, *per se*. Rather, the subject of consideration is the type of pain that arises from disease, injury, or illness; that is, pain that has a root cause in the body of a person (Twycross and Lack, 1983). The pain in question may not terminate in the

157

K.Wm. Wildes (ed.), Birth, Suffering and Death, 157–169.
© 1992 *Kluwer Academic Publishers. Printed in the Netherlands.*

body, thus the physical pain may give rise to spiritual or emotional pain, but the fundamental cause of the pain under consideration is the physiological system of the person. The Association of the Study of Pain defines this type of pain as: "An unpleasant sensory or emotional experience associated with actual or potential tissue damage as described in terms of such damage" (Associated for Study of Pain, 1980).

Pain relief may involve anything from an aspirin to morphine. Aspirin and other non-opioid medications are given to relieve minor pains. Usually, there are no ethical problems arising from the use of these medications because there are few serious side effects. True, a person may become addicted to the use of minor pain medication, but addiction does not arise from the mere use of pain relief.

In itself pain relief is a beneficial action; one of the principle means people have for caring for one another. Therefore, if proximate or long term injury does not result from the effort to relieve pain, ethical problems are not associated with pain relief. The use of opioid drugs however; that is, drugs which remove pain by repressing the activity of the central nervous system, does present a problem because of their proximate and long term effects. Opioid analgesics are either weak, such as codeine, or strong, such as morphine. While codeine does not have extensive side effects, morphine may impair cognitive function. Given in larger quantities, morphine may sedate a person to the extent that he or she loses consciousness. Such large doses may also repress the central nervous system and thus hasten death by making it difficult to breath (Bonica, 1990). Insofar as the use of strong opioids is concerned, such as morphine or morphine sulfate, it is difficult to predict accurately how they will affect people. Each patient is different insofar as tolerance of pain is concerned and insofar as reaction to morphine is concerned (Kaiko et al., 1986; Vertafridda et al., 1987). Hence, it is erroneous to generalize and maintain that the ethical issues under discussion arise every time morphine is used to quell pain. Sometimes even severe pain may be relieved sufficiently without the cognitive function of the patient being impaired significantly, or for long periods of time (Twycross and Lack, 1983). However, sometimes the very purpose of the pain medication is to render the patient comatose as death approaches (Hyers et al., 1986); for example, Schneiderman and Spragg maintain: "If the decision is made to end the use of mechanical ventilation in a patient whose life depends on it, all participants in the decision should realize that the patient's death will follow. We believe it is important to medicate such patients before ventilation is withdrawn to eliminate the discomfort of agonal efforts to breath. As an unavoidable side effect of the medication, survival may be shortened by minutes or hours" (Schneiderman and Spragg, 1988). If the use of pain medication either impairs the cognitive function of the patient or hastens death, why would this present a problem as long as the pain is relieved? There are two reasons for concern; both drawn from the teaching of the Church in regard to stewardship of life.

1. In the Catholic tradition, acceptance of suffering, of which physical pain is a prototype, is a means to spiritual growth. "The joy and the suffering of this life have a Christian meaning; its joys are signs of the hope for everlasting life in his kingdom, which is already present here on earth in promise; and its sorrows are a sharing in his cross through which a victorious resurrection is to be achieved" (Pope John Paul II, 1984). "Suffering, especially suffering during the last moments of life, has a special place in God's saving plan: it is in fact a sharing in Christ's passion and a union with the redeeming sacrifice which he offered in obedience to the Father's will" (Congregation for Doctrine of the Faith, 1975).

Clearly, if as a result of the medication to alleviate pain, the patient is unable to think clearly, or lapses into a coma, there will be reduced opportunity to "share in the sufferings of Christ". Thus, the opportunity for expiation of the guilt of sin and for spiritual progress may be lost.

2. The second concern arises from the use of strong opioid pain relief is that hastening death is often "an act of euthanasia" (Congregation for Doctrine of the Faith, 1975). Is hastening death through the use of pain medication an act of euthanasia or is there another explanation in keeping with the teaching of the Church?

II. THE TEACHING OF THE CATHOLIC CHURCH

1. Teaching in Regard to Maintaining Consciousness

The teaching of the Catholic Church is always realistic and compassionate when applied to particular cases. Thus, while the Church presents the ideal that suffering may be a way of joining oneself more closely to the sufferings of Christ, it also states: "It would be imprudent to impose a heroic way of acting as a general rule. Hence, human and Christian prudence suggest for the majority of sick people the use of medicine capable of alleviating and suppressing pain, even those that may cause as secondary effect, semi-consciousness and reduced lucidity. As for those who are unable to express themselves, one can reasonably presume that they wish to take those pain killers and have them administered according to the doctor's advice" (Congregation for Doctrine of the Faith, 1975).

Though certain assumptions may be made when caring for incapacitated patients, patients who are capable of making health care decisions for themselves should be consulted before pain medication is given. Insofar as possible, a person imbued with the Catholic faith may prefer "to moderate the use of pain killers, in order to accept voluntarily at least part of their sufferings and thus associate themselves in a conscious way with the suffering of Christ" (Congregation for Doctrine of the Faith, 1975). Hence, no blanket judgments should be made that would treat all patients indiscriminately insofar as pain relief is concerned. Knowing that the capacity to endure pain differs from one person to another, pain relief should be provided in such a way as to enable each person to fulfill personal and family obligations. For example, as death approaches the patient should be fortified with fitting spiritual consolation. The Sacraments of Reconciliation, Anointing, and Eucharist are more effectively received if a person is conscious and aware. However, if the pain cannot be relieved unless the patient is sedated to the point of unconsciousness, this would be an accepted form of therapy. "We are not obliged to think that all pain must be endured at any price or that socially one must not attempt to reduce and calm patients" (Pontifical Council, Cor Unum, 1989).

When using pain medication, it must be clear that the purpose is to relieve suffering and anxiety on the part of the patient, not to save the medical staff from physical labor, nor to save the family from emotional strain as a loved one nears death (Pontifical Council, Cor Unum, 1980). The good of the patient must be paramount. When considering the use of pain medication, recent surveys indicate that over medication often is utilized in nursing homes as a means of "controlling" patients (Goldber, 1987). The same attitude may lead to over medication as death approaches.

Helping the patient to be conscious as death approaches may seem to some to be unnecessary and even brutal. But for the person of faith, death is the last loving act, not a penalty to be grudgingly endured. Catholic teaching does not present suffering or death as a human good but rather as an inevitable event which may be transformed into a moral good if accepted as a way of identifying more closely with Christ. Nor should the acceptance of suffering and death be considered a passive process. In their attempt to specify more clearly what it means to suffer and die, modern theologians have concentrated on death as a personal act of a human being, an act that terminates earthly existence but also fulfills it (Congregation for Doctrine of the Faith, 1975). Thus the person is not merely passive in the face of death, and death is different for the just than for the sinner. In the view of Karl Rahner (1965), a view accepted and developed by many theologians, death is an active consummation, a maturing self-realization that embodies what each person has made of himself or herself during life. Death becomes a ratification of life, not merely an inevitable process. It is an event, an action in which the freedom of the person is intimately involved. Dying with Christ is an adventure; it is a consequence of, but not a condemnation for, sin. This is a new approach to death, yet it is thoroughly in keeping with the Christian tradition. Indeed, this view of death seems to describe more clearly the experience of Christ, who offered his life rather than have it taken from him, who completed his love and generosity in the final act of obedience to the Father: "It is consummated" (Jn 19: 30).

As death approaches then, narcotics may relieve pain, but narcotics do not help people prepare for the act of death. Only the presence of loving caregivers and family members make possible the act of death in a Christian manner. "What is therefore important, is to protect vigorously against any systematic plunging into unconsciousness of the fatally ill, and to demand on the contrary, that medical and nursing personnel learn how to listen to the dying" (Pontifical Council, *Cor Unum*, 1980).

In sum, the teaching of the Catholic Church in regard to the use of pain medication which may impair cognitive function is expressed aptly by Pope Pius XII. When asked by anesthesiologists: "May narcotics be used at the approach of death even if the use of narcotics may shorten life?" he responded: "If no other means exist, and if, in the given circumstances, this does not prevent the carrying out of other religious and moral duties: Yes. In this case, of course, death is in no way intended or sought, even if the risk of it is reasonably taken; the intention is simply to relieve pain effectively, using for this purpose painkillers available to medicine" (Congregation for Doctrine of the Faith, 1980). In this statement, Pius XII indicates that the principle of double effect underlies the teaching of the Church in regard to the use of pain medication. We shall study this principle in more detail in Section III.

2. Teaching in Regard to Hastening Death

Ethical confusion occurs more often in regard to the proper treatment of persons approaching death than in any other phase of patient care. Some physicians and theologians and lawyers wish to prolong life unless death is inevitable and unavoidable. Thus, even life without the potential for cognitive function must be prolonged as long as possible (May *et al.*, 1990). For some hastening death even as a result of pain relief is morally unacceptable. Others believe that using pain medication with the risk of impeding respiration and thereby hastening death is "passive euthanasia" (Goldber, 1987). Still others, thinking that medicine has no intrinsic goods or values, tend to refer all decisions concerning "hastening death" to families of the patient, or what is worse, to the courts (Robinson and Horan, 1987).

In order to understand clearly Church teaching in regard to the difference between intending to hasten death (euthanasia) and intending to relieve pain even if death occurs more swiftly, certain distinctions must be considered briefly.

a. Human life is a gift from God, "bestowed in order to accomplish a mission. Thus the right to life is not of foremost importance, but rather directing oneself toward the end of perfecting oneself according to God's plan" (Pontifical Council, *Cor Unum*, 1980).

Human beings have been called to make their lives useful, but they may not destroy life at their own will. Murder and suicide are contrary to God's providence for human beings. However, because our mission in life is to love God, love ourselves and love our neighbor, a person need not take positive actions to prolong human life at all costs. "A person's duty is to care for his body, his functions, its organs; to do everything he can to render himself capable of attaining to God". This duty implies giving up things which " of themselves may be good" (Pontifical Council, *Cor Unum*, 1980).

In Catholic teaching then, one has a moral obligation to eschew murder and suicide because these actions bespeak a power over human life which in God's Providence is not given to human beings. However, insofar as taking positive steps to prolong life is concerned, a person should not prolong life if prolonging life would interfere with the person's mission in life. In Catholic tradition the moral obligation to prolong life is usually expressed by saying that when faced with a fatal pathology, one should use the means to prolong life, unless these means impose a grave burden upon the patient or the therapy is futile. If the therapy which would prolong life imposes a grave burden or is futile, then there is no moral obligation to use it.

b. In Catholic teaching, euthanasia is an action or omission which of itself or by intention causes death, in order that suffering may be eliminated (Congregation for Doctrine of the Faith, 1975). Euthanasia may be *voluntary* or *involuntary*; depending on the desire of the person who dies. Voluntary euthanasia involves suicide on the part of the patient and assisted suicide on the part of the care giver. Euthanasia may be *active* or *passive*. Euthanasia is active if the cause of death is induced, (e.g., gunshot, poison). Active euthanasia is prohibited because it involves the direct killing of an innocent person. Euthanasia is *passive* if the cause of death is present in a person's body but is not resisted when there is a moral obligation to do so. Hence, passive euthanasia occurs when a person with a fatal pathology is allowed to die even though therapy to cure the illness would not impose a grave burden or be ineffective. Passive euthanasia is ethically unacceptable because it intends the death of another (by omitting acts) when there is a moral obligation to prolong the life of the person in question.

A prominent example of the confusion existing in regard to the distinction between passive euthanasia (intending death by withholding therapy from a person with a fatal pathology) and withholding therapy from a person with a fatal pathology because the therapy would be burdensome or useless occurred in the case of Baby Doe in Indiana (Pless, 1983). Baby Doe was a child with Down Syndrome suffering from duodenal atresia. Without a simple surgery, he would die due to an inability to ingest food and to receive nourishment. Would the surgery impose a grave burden on Baby Doe? No, because it is a surgery performed on normal children all the time and never thought to be a grave burden. Would the surgery have been effective? It seems so because it would have enabled Baby Doe to pursue his purpose in life. Down Syndrome children may be impaired but they are able to know, love and relate to others. However, Baby Doe was not given the life prolonging therapy. His parents, aided by a court order, maintained that withholding care from the infant was not euthanasia because it did not directly cause his death. Rather he would die of the underlying pathology. But the parents and the court were in error as they considered whether or not to prolong the life of Baby Doe. Because the surgery did not constitute a grave burden and was not futile, it should have been performed. In sum, the direct intention of the parents was to hasten Baby Doe's death, not to avoid useless or burdensome therapy.

There is a significant moral difference between euthanasia, either active or passive, and using pain medication with the direct intention of alleviating pain as death approaches. Even if the pain medication hastens death for a dying person, if the direct intention of the act is to remove pain, then hastening death is an accidental side effect. In euthanasia the intention is to cause death in order to relieve pain. Even in face of severe suffering the intention to take the life of another is not in accord with the providence of God. However, the intention of removing pain from a dying person is within the providence of God. If the death of the person is hastened, by reason of the fact that strong pain medication is used, it is an undesired side effect. If there were therapy which would remove the pain without hastening death, such a therapy would be utilized (Congregation for Doctrine of the Faith, 1975; Pope Pius XII, 1984).

Notice that when stating the teaching of the Church in regard to pain relief, it is not enough to state that pain relief may be utilized even if a side effect is to hasten the death of the patient. Rather, the statement must be more specific; the teaching of the Church is conveyed accurately only if the moribund condition of the patient is stated (Congregation for Doctrine of the Faith, 1975). The need to limit the hastening of death by pain medication only to the moribund is clear from the following example. A young man breaks a leg while skiing and is in serious pain from the injury and the surgery necessary to mend the compound fracture. The amount of pain medication necessary to relieve the pain would seriously impair respiratory function. The risk associated with this much pain medication would not be proportionate to the overall well-being of the patient. In the case of a person who will die soon however, provided there are no spiritual or family obligations to be fulfilled, there is no great benefit to extending the person's life for a few hours or days. Thus, pain medication, even if it would hasten death, could be utilized when there is no moral obligation to prolong life.

A growing number of physicians and medical ethicists speak out in favor of euthanasia either active or passive (Angell, 1988; Wanzer, 1987). Some maintain that active euthanasia or suicide is the ultimate act of the autonomous person (Humphry et al., 1988). Some of these proponents of euthanasia are confused, either about the criteria which allow withholding or withdrawal of life support or about the ethical use of pain medication at the time of death (Humphry, 1986). Others however, simply deny the consistent and customary teaching of medical ethics and religion. In the Netherlands for example, euthanasia is tolerated by the legal system (Welie, 1989). In the face of these actions and allegations the teaching of the Catholic Church has been reiterated (Congregation for Doctrine of the Faith, 1975): "It may happen that, by reason of prolonged and barely tolerable pain, for deeply personal or other reasons, people may be led to believe that they can legitimately ask for death or obtain it for others. Although in these cases the guilt of the individual may be reduced or completely absent, nevertheless the error of judgment into which the conscience falls, perhaps in good faith, does not change the nature of this act of killing, which will always be in itself something to be rejected".

In sum, the teaching of the Catholic Church clearly renounces euthanasia, whether active or passive, but does allow the use of pain medication which hastens death if there is no moral obligation to prolong the life of the suffering person. "Human and Christian prudence suggests for the majority of sick people the use of medicines capable of alleviating or suppressing pain even though these may cause as a secondary effect of semi-consciousness and reduced lucidity" (Congregation for Doctrine of the Faith, 1975). In this case of course, death is in no way intended or sought, even if the risk of it is reasonably taken, the intention is simply to relieve pain effectively". Once again, the Church bases its teaching in this regard upon the principle of double effect. In order to understand Church teaching more fully, a word must be said about this principle.

III. PRINCIPLE OF DOUBLE EFFECT

In human life, pursuing a desirable and worthwhile good may involve accepting some unwanted side effects. When seeking to be rid of an inflamed appendix, one must accept the pain and discomfort of surgery; when defending oneself from an attack, one may inflict injury upon another person even though the defender has no desire to injure another person. In general, actions of this nature are ethically analyzed by using the principle of double effect. Briefly this principle states (Boyle, 1980):

When a desired effect and an undesired effect result from a human act, the act is morally good only if four conditions are fulfilled:

a) the object of the act itself must be morally good; that is, the effect of the act in the moral order contributes to the overall well-being of

the person who chooses the act;
b)   only the good results of the act may be intended;
c)   the good effect must not result from the bad effect;
d)   there must be a proportionately good reason for permitting the bad
      effect.

As we shall see later, the last three criteria are used to verify the first criterion: that the object of the act is morally good (Connery, 1981).

In the two cases we have studied in this essay, relieving severe pain in such a way that a comatose condition is induced or death is hastened, it is clear that both actions are acceptable only if the intention of the care giver is morally good; namely, to relieve pain. But the good intention alone does not justify the action. There must also be judgment that the un-wanted effect is not so detrimental to the person that it violates the good effect which is desired. That is the meaning of the fourth criterion: "There must be a proportion between the desired effect and undesired effect". Thus, it would be unethical to give a patient in pain, who will recover from his illness, a heavy dose of morphine sulfate which might hasten death, even though the same dose could be given a moribund person, (cf. example p. 163). The proportion between the good and the evil effects is not verified in the case of the person who it is hoped will recover. Simply because the act accomplishes something good (the relief of pain) does not imply that one is then free from moral discernment concerning the unwanted effects of the action. Forming a morally good intention involves an analysis, based upon objective reality, of the relationship between the desired and undesired effect. This is all encompassed in the effort to analyze the moral object of the act.

Another method of understanding the principle of double effect is to realize that the unwanted effect would not be allowed, were it not connected necessarily with achieving the desired effect. Thus, if there were another method of relieving pain, a method which did not involve the undesirable side effect of putting the patient in a coma or risking an earlier death, then the more benign method should be chosen. At present, development of a pain medication to relieve severe pain that does not affect the central nervous system is unlikely (Hyers et al., 1986). Hence, the potential undesirable side effects of relief for severe pain will be present for the foreseeable future.

The most authoritative secular voice on medical ethics in our pluralistic society, The President's Commission for Ethics in Medicine and Research, agrees in substance with the theology of Catholic tradition when discussing the problem of pain relief and the risk of death that may result from the use of pain medication. For example, the Commission states (President's Commission, 1983):

a. "Were a patient experiencing great pain from a condition that will be cured in a few days, use of morphine at doses that would probably lead to death by inducing respiratory depression would usually be unacceptable".

b. "For a patient in great pain, especially from a condition that has proved to be untreatable and is expected to be rapidly fatal – morphine can be both morally and legally acceptable if pain relief cannot be achieved by less risky means".

The Commission however, in offering solutions for the problem of the use of pain medication is reluctant to endorse the principle of double effect. While "[T]he Commission makes use of many of the moral considerations found in the doctrine" it believes that "the moral issue is whether or not the decision makers have considered the full range of foreseeable effects ... and have found the risks to be justified" (President's Commission, 1983).

However, analysis of the risks, and whether or not they are justified, is precisely the meaning of the first criterion of the principle of double effect. To put it another way, the determination that an act is morally good, must be made in light of the object of the act; this implies that all the significant circumstances are considered as one determines the object of the act. At times, one of the circumstances may be an essential part of the moral object, e.g., defacing a cup is morally different than defacing a cup which is a chalice. The Commission, especially in the example it uses when considering the first criterion, (i.e., "administering a pain killer") (President's Commission, 1983) considers the moral act in the abstract, apart from its circumstances. All significant circumstances must be considered when discerning the moral object of the act. (Administering a pain killer *to whom; what* is the physical condition of the person to whom it is administered?).

The misconception of The Commission points out the complexity of the principle of double effect. Many times it is used as an extrinsic and *apriori* tool to solve moral problems. Actually, it is more accurate to conceive of it as a conclusion drawn from an objective and thorough analysis of the moral act in question; that is, an analysis of the moral object and circumstances. This type of objective analysis is not complete unless the condition of the patient and the risks resulting from a proposed therapy are considered beforehand.

CONCLUSION

The teaching of the Church in regard to pain relief, especially as death approaches is most important in contemporary society because of the campaign to approve and legalize euthanasia. There is no doubt that euthanasia, whether passive or active, has an attraction for people imbued with pragmatic, consequentialist and cost-effective philosophies of life. But these philosophies are short sighted. In the long run they betray human dignity and the bonds of community. On the other hand, the teaching of the Church presents a deeper and transcendent appreciation of the human person in community. Only if the human dignity of persons in pain is respected will they receive pain relief in accord with their mission in life. The teaching of the Church in conjunction with the practice of ethical physicians, gives hope for the future insofar as care of the sick and dying is concerned.

BIBLIOGRAPHY

American Association of Retired Persons: (1986), *Elder Abuse Project*, Washington, DC.
Angell, M.: 1988, 'Euthanasia', *The New England Journal of Medicine* 319 (20), 1348–1350.
Associated for Study of Pain (I.S.A.P.): 1980, 'Pain terms: A list with definitions and notes on usage' *Pain*, 8, 249–252.
Bonica, J.: 1990, 'History of pain concepts and therapies', in Bonica, J. (ed.), *The Management of Pain*, Len and Febiger, Philadelphia, pp. 2–18.
Boyle, J.: 1980, 'Toward understanding the principle of double effect', (*90*) *Ethics*, 527.
Congregation for Doctrine of the Faith: 1975, 'The reality of life after death', in Flannery, A. (ed.), 1982 *Vatican Council II: More Documents*, Costello, New York, pp. 500–504.
Congregation for Doctrine of the Faith: 1980, *Declaration on Euthanasia*, United States Catholic Conference, Washington, D. C., 6.
Connery, J.: 1981, 'Catholic ethics, has the norm for role making changed?' *Theological Studies*, 42(2), 232–250.
Goldber, R.: 1987, 'The right to die: The case for and against passive euthanasia', *Disability Handicap and Society*, 2(1) 21–39.
Humphry, D.: 1986, *The Right to Die: Understanding Euthanasia*, Harper & Row, New York.
Humphry, D., *et al.*: 1988, 'Aid in dying: The right to die or the right to kill – a public

forum', *International Review of Natural Family Planning.*

Hyers, T., *et al.*: 1986, 'Withholding and withdrawing ventilations', *American Review of Respiratory Distress*, 143(6), 1327–1331.

Kaiko, R. *et al.*: 1986, 'Clinical Analgesic Studies and Sources of Variation in Analgesic Responses to Morphine', in Foley, K., Inturrisi, C. (eds.), *Opioid Analgesics in the Management of Clinical Pain*, Raven Press, New York, pp. 14–24.

Loeser, J. and Kelly, J. (eds.): 1989, *Managing the Chronic Pain Patient: Theory and Practice at the University of Washington Multidisciplinary Pain Center*, Raven Press, New York.

May, W., *et al.*: 1990, 'Criteria for withholding and withdrawing treatment', *Linacre Quarterly*, v.5:7 n.3, p.81.

Pitman, B. F.: 1990, 'Approaches to palliative care: Notes of a death watcher', in Foley, K, Bionca, J. (eds.), *Proceedings of the Second International Congress on Cancer Pain*, Raven Press, New York, pp. 393–397.

Pless, J.: 1983, 'The story of baby doe', *The New England Journal of Medicine*, 309, 604.

Pontifical Council: 1980, *Cor Unum*, 'Questions of ethics regarding fatally ill and the dying', in K. O'Rourke and P. Boyle (eds.), 1989, *Medical Ethics: Sources of Catholic Teaching*, CHA, 219, 305.

Pope John Paul II: 1984, 'The Christian Meaning of Suffering', in *Origins*, 13, 609–619.

Pope Pius XII: 1944, 'Christian principles of the medical profession', in O'Rourke, K. and Boyle, P. (eds.), 1989, *Medical Ethics Sources of Catholic Teaching*, CHA, pp. 217–302.

Pope Pius XII: 1957, 'Address to Anesthesiologists', in O'Rourke, K. and Boyle, P. (eds.), 1989, *Medical Ethics Sources of Catholic Teaching*, CHA, pp. 217–302.

President's Commission for the Study of Ethical Problems in Medicine and Biomedical and Behavioral Research: 1983, *Deciding to Forego Life-Sustaining Treatment*, U.S. Government Printing Office, 80.

Rahner, K.: 1965, *On the Theology of Death*, Herder and Herder, New York.

Robinson, R. and Horan, D: 1987, 'Termination of medical treatment: Imminent legislative issues', *Catholic Lawyer*, 31(2) 99–11.

Schneiderman, L. J. and Spragg, R.: 1988, 'Ethical decisions in discontinuing mechanical ventilation', *The New England Journal of Medicine*, 318(5) 984–988.

Twycross, R. and Lack, S.: 1983, *Symptom Control in Far Advanced Cancer: Pain Relief*, Melbourne.

Vertafridda, V. *et al.*: 1987, 'A validation study of the WHO method for cancer pain relief', *Cancer*, 59 n.4, 850–856.

Wanzer, S. *et al.*: 1989, 'The physicians' responsibility toward hopelessly ill patients', *The New England Journal of Medicine*, 320(13) 844–849.

Welie, J: 1989, 'Euthanasia in the Netherlands', unpublished article.

THOMAS J. BOLE, III

WHY ALMOST ANY COST TO OTHERS TO PRESERVE THE LIFE OF THE IRREVERSIBLY COMATOSE CONSTITUTES AN EXTRAORDINARY BURDEN

Prominent Roman Catholic thinkers have recently argued (Boyle, 1991; Grisez, 1990; May, 1990) that one is obligated to provide food and water to irreversibly comatose patients, i.e., those in a permanently vegetative state (hereinafter: PVS). Food and water are normally considered "ordinary", ordinate, means to preserve human life, and one is normally obligated to preserve one's own life and those of any patient in one's charge by providing nutrition. Patients in PVS, however, are unable to swallow, and the nutrition has to be provided through a feeding tube inserted into the stomach. These thinkers deny that the invasiveness makes the provision of nutrition "extraordinary", or non-obligatory. They think that, if one were not obligated to provide patients in PVS with food and water, one would face a morally unacceptable dilemma. Either one would be forced to choose a means to save the costs (not simply of artificially feeding the patient, but of overall care) that is homicidal, since it is effective only if the patient dies. Or one would have to refuse care in general, "which is tantamount to abandoning the patient", and this "is generally difficult to justify, and for wealthy societies sets a dangerously unjust precedent" (Boyle, 1991, p. 17; cf. Grisez, 1990). It may be that an individual or a family is so strapped financially as to make it extraordinary, and thus non-obligatory, to bear the costs of preserving the life of the patient in PVS. Affluent societies such as that of the United States, however, ought to underwrite such costs where necessary. Otherwise, such a society would be denying that a person's life is an intrinsic, non-instrumental good. It would be committed to an untenable dualism between the human person, i.e., a human being with full moral standing, and that human's life[1], so that in the ultimate cases of human lives incapable of any potentiality for spiritual function, as in patients in PVS, and in the cases of severely mentally handicapped as well, society would consider life intrinsically worthless.[2]

These contentions highlight two issues that the advent of expensive life-sustaining technology raises. First, what sort of good is constituted by human life without potential for conscious, or spiritual, function, and

171

K.Wm. Wildes (ed.), Birth, Suffering and Death, 171–187.
© 1992 *Kluwer Academic Publishers. Printed in the Netherlands.*

what sort of obligation do others who ought to care for someone have if that individual has such a life? More specifically, what sort of obligation do these others have to preserve such life rather than to pursue other intrinsically choiceworthy goods, whether Christian salvation, or the non-religious goods of supporting art, or good food and fellowship, or life capable of regaining some conscious function? Given finite resources, efforts to preserve these lives usually inhibits the pursuit of other goods. Second, to what extent are others obligated to pursue that good at the expense of other pursuits? Even if we assume that there is an obligation to preserve artificially the lives of patients in PVS, at what point is this obligation defeasible by the costs that its fulfillment would impose? This is in fact two questions. There is a question of individual morality, namely, of what costs other moral agents who should be concerned with the patient in PVS are obligated to bear, and of what costs would defeat this obligation. And there is a question of public morality, namely, of costs that the body politic (in an affluent and secular pluralist society such as the United States) ought to bear, and of costs that would defeat the obligation. Proponents of tube feeding patients in PVS assume that the body politic (at least in the United States) has a moral obligation to underwrite these costs. But even if one grants that the good of life obligates those who ought to care for such a patient to nourish him, it does not follow that the state in a secular pluralist society ought to underwrite this care.

In what follows I first review the ordinary-extraordinary distinction, because it embodies the clearest and most comprehensive set of reflections available upon what sorts of means are and are not ordinate, and therefore obligatory, to save human life. I then make five contentions. First, the lack of obvious benefit, whether in improved health or even in sustaining a life that the patient can positively value, seems to make any costs involved in artificially preserving the life of patients in PVS extraordinary, and therefore non-obligatory. Second, for those obligated to care for such a patient, it would seems appropriate to allow that patient to die in dignity, i.e., to provide hygienic (and perhaps cosmetic) care. Accordingly, any costs other than those of hygienic care while the patient expires would be extraordinary, because inappropriate. One may, of course, have the contrary intuition, that preservative care is appropriate, rather than hygienic care alone. However, proponents of this contrary intuition do not, I contend, bear the burden of proving that it should be normative even for those who disagree. Third, in order to show that the public purse ought to help underwrite the costs of preserving the lives of patients in PVS, one must show that the preservation of such lives is normative for the common welfare in a secular and pluralist. Even if one can show that those who have an obligation to care for such patients ought to preserve their lives, it does not follow that such an obligation falls upon the body politic. The upshot of these contentions is to show that, even if the life of patients in PVS is intrinsically good, it does not follow that one is obligated to shoulder any costs to preserve it.

The final two contentions turn to the type of good that life might be. The fourth contention is that, in non-sectarian terms, the life of a human in PVS is not an intrinsic good that ought to be preserved artificially, in clear contrast to the life of a human person. This contrast between human being and human person is foreign to the Christian tradition. My last contention, however, is that, even if we accept as part of Christian revelation that God makes each instance of a human being intrinsically good, i.e., not to be used as a mere means, this good is fundamentally distorted when the life of a patient in PVS is preserved by invasive means such as tube feeding, rather than being allowed to expire with due dignity, and with prayers for the patient's salvation in Christ.

I

Crucial both to my contentions and to those who defend the obligation of preserving the lives of patients in PVS by tube feeding, is the traditional Roman Catholic distinction between ordinary and extraordinary means of preserving life. The distinction arose 400 years ago, in a period perceived as one of great scientific and medical advances. Vesalius' *De humani corporis fabrica* (1563) had put anatomy on a scientific basis, and Descartes was certain that medicine's progress would allow him to live for over 100 years, rather than the 49 he lived in fact.[3] Therapeutic approaches were costly, however, and not only in monetary terms, as surgery without the benefit of anesthesia or antibiotics makes us realize. Was one always obligated to accept such treatment, if it might save his life, lest refusal might be tantamount to suicide?

Roman Catholic theologians at the time answered by distinguishing between obligatory means and non-obligatory means to preserve one's life.[4] Only ordinary means could be obligatory. Extraordinary means endanger the moral life of the patient and of others because they are intemperate, i.e., they do not usually leave sufficient room to satisfy other goods, the goods that give life value.

The tradition isolated three factors, any of which alone or in combination may render treatment to preserve life extraordinary and therefore non-obligatory: (1) difficulty of availability, i.e., access only by hard-to-obtain [*exquisitis*] means, (2) excessive burden, and (3) insufficient *spes salutis*, i.e., expectation of health or of a (relatively) sound life. The point of the distinction was to keep in mind that, given the plurality of intrinsic goods which a Christian must be aware of, and given that the Christian's paramount concern is the spiritual good of his eternal salvation, the good of preserving human life should not be pursued intemperately, i.e., in a manner so as to hinder significantly his obligations to other goods, especially that of eternal salvation. Moreover, the abovementioned factors were not meant to be analytically exhaustive, or even exclusive; the tradition within which the distinction arose was casuist, based upon case-by-case analysis, of which the factors give rough summaries. From this angle one can see that the first factor can perhaps be collapsed into the second. In any case, the second and third factors are the crucial ones, because they each contain several significant kinds.

The burdens that render means to preserve life extraordinary can be financially excessive, if they impose what the tradition calls a *sumptus extraordinarius* (i.e., an inordinate cost) or *media pretiosa* (i.e., extravagant means). Burdens can also be excessive physically, in the sense of imposing too much pain or suffering (the tradition speaks of *quidam cruciatus*, considerable torture, or *ingens dolor*, immoderate grief), or excessive psychologically, imposing means that are repulsive (and thus elicit a *vehemens horror*, in the graphic phrasing of the tradition, i.e., a violent quaking or ardent repulsion).[5] In addition, burdens can be excessive in the sense of requiring great effort (*summus labor*), or imposing too much indignity (*nimia dura*), as life severely maimed or dysfunctional might bring.

Of immediate relevance is that excessively burdensome means to preserve life may be burdensome not only to the patient, but also relevant others. This is implied in the remarks of Pope Pius XII in his 1957 address to a congress of anesthesiologists, an address that explicitly appeals to the ordinary-extraordinary distinction: "[N]ormally one is held to use only ordinary means [to prolong life] – according to the circumstances of persons, places, times, and culture – that is to say, means that do not involve any grave burden for oneself or another" (1957, p. 1030). That others may also be excessively burdened is more explicit in the "Declaration on Euthanasia" issued by the Congregation for the Doctrine of the Faith in 1980:

[O]ne cannot impose on anyone the obligation to have recourse to a technique which is already in use but which carries a risk or is burdensome. Such a refusal is not the equivalent of suicide; on the contrary, it should be considered as an acceptance of the human condition, or a wish to avoid the application of a medical procedure dispropor-tionate to the results which can be expected, or a desire not to impose excessive expense on the family or community (p. 295).

Although the citation's point of view is the patient's, the reasons given are meant to be intersubjectively valid. They can therefore be validly invoked by others beside the patient, and in this case one would also have weigh them against whatever obligations those others might have to the patient. Relevant others are not only those who would normally be obligated to care for the patient, e.g., relatives or healthcare professionals; they would also be third parties, whether public or private, who are significantly underwriting the patient's treatment. Third-party payers are especially worth keeping in mind inasmuch as the explosion of effective medical life-saving technology since 1960 has been accompanied by an expansion of the percent of total healthcare costs borne by third-party payers from 51% to 74% in 1988 (Office of National Cost Estimates, 1990, p. 3). The relevance of this expansion for care of the irreversibly comatose will concern us in the next section.

First, however, the third factor of the distinction between ordinary and extraordinary care should be explicated, the factor of *spes salutis*, a reasonable expectation of life or health. "Life", it is important to note, means a life capable of existing on its own, and this implies a life apart from a permanent and uninterrupted dependence upon invasive proce-dures, whether they be feeding tubes or more elaborate machines. The point is not that such interventions were not available when the notion of *spes salutis* was formulated, but that a life of such dependence is by definition not what *salus* means.

Spes salutis covers a number of distinctive considerations. There is insufficient *spes salutis* if there is too low a probability of success of the means of preserving life. Even if there is sufficient probability that the means will succeed in preserving life, there is still insufficient *spes salutis* if the resulting life is of too poor a quality. Moreover, even if the means will probably succeed and yield a life of acceptable quality, there is insufficient *spes salutis* if there is too meager a quantity of life. A reasonable expectation of life or health, then, covers not only a sufficient probability that the means will be successful, but also that the result will be a life of sufficient quality and of sufficient quantity. Given this explication of the ordinary-extraordinary distinction, is the preservation of life of the irreversibly comatose by artificial nutrition and hydration ordinary, and therefore obligatory, or is it extraordinary?

II

A. Lack of Spes Salutis For Patients In PVS Makes Efforts To Preserve Their Lives Extraordinary

My first contention is that any of the costs involved in artificially preserving the lives of patients in PVS are extraordinary, and so non-obligatory, because they provide no *spes salutis*, no reasonable expectation either of health or of a life that can in any way be positively valued by the patient. This contention takes it as evident that *spes salutis* means a reasonable expectation of benefit.[6] The ordinary-extraordinary distinction is based upon the usual judgment of men about appropriate means in the circumstances; the distinction is a casuistic one. It is the usual judgment of men that preserving human life no longer capable of any conscious feeling or function, is not beneficial.[7] In the words of the theological opinion of the Diocese of Providence as it ruled that artificial nutrition and hydration could be removed from a patient in PVS: "[T]he medical treatments which are being provided the patient, even those which are supplying nutrition and hydration artificially, offer no reasonable hope of benefit to her. This lack of reasonable hope of benefit renders <them> ... futile and thus extraordinary".[8] Any costs, whether economic or psychological or physical, to preserve the life of such a patient would therefore be extraordinary, because they would be futile.

B. The Care Appropriate For Patients In PVS Is Not Preserving Their Lives, But Letting Them Die With Dignity

One might object that I have begged the question at issue, namely, whether preservation of human life, even if incapable of any function other than the merely biological, is worthwhile by itself. Accordingly, "faithfully caring for comatose persons benefits them not only by sustaining their lives but by maintaining a moral bond of human solidarity with them" (Grisez, 1990, p. 40). *Sed contra*, my second contention is that appropriate care for patients in PVS is to provide what hygienic (and possibly cosmetic) care is requisite to allow their lives to reach their natural termination in a dignified manner.

There are two reasons why this care, and not tube feeding, would be obligatory upon those who should provide care for such a patient. The first is that the only possible benefit that can be given to such a patient is that which allows the life to end in a way that shows respect to its possessor. To ensure hygienic (and perhaps cosmetic) care seems sufficient to show this respect. By contrast, there is no possible benefit to an irreversibly comatose patient by tube feeding, because the patient cannot revive; one is only delaying the inevitable. Moreover, to prolong life artificially that is incapable of in any way appreciating the effort, is tantamount not to "maintaining a moral bond of human solidarity", but to giving inappropriate care, care that artificially delays the patient's death for no good reason. Such care denies the patient's humanity by belying the fact that finitude is part of human life. A moral bond of human solidarity is better shown by ensuring that the patient's life reaches its natural end in a dignified manner. If this reason is good, the conclusion of the first contention is reaffirmed: any cost involved in preserving the life of a patient in PVS is extraordinary, because inappropriate.

The second reason that, even if tube feeding such patients were the morally most appropriate course of action, it would be so only within the framework of overall maintenance care, and such care requires too much money and/or effort for most. $110,000 per year is required to preserve artificially a patient in PVS.[9] Moreover, the fact that most such patients are preserved in health care institutions suggests very strongly that the effort to care for them at home is too great. Even if the costs of tube feeding alone are but a small percentage of the total cost caring for that patient[10], the logic of tube feeding commits one to a course of care that is so burdensome that it cannot be obligatory. If it were so, one would be obligated to preserving life incapable of any spirituality at grave costs to the pursuit of any of the manifestations of the life of the spirit. This consequence is a clear violation of the notion that the means to preserve merely biological human life should not endanger the pursuit of the spiritual values to which such life is properly ordained. Since the overall cost of tube feeding and otherwise maintaining a patient in PVS is extraordinarily burdensome for most (even if this maintenance were the ideal course of action), then most of those who are obligated to care for such patients are obligated only to ensure that they die in dignity.

C. The Obligation To Preserve the Lives of Patients In PVS (If It Exists At All) Is Not a Political Obligation

Those who think it morally obligatory to tube feed patients in PVS, would grant that the total financial burden involved in doing so is extraordinary for most families. They assume, however, that preserving such life is not extraordinary, hence that it is obligatory, for third-party payers in general, and in particular for the public purse of affluent societies such as that of the United States: "[I]f the overall costs of treatment are the burden one wishes to avoid,the level at which the burdens become disproportionate is very high. For avoiding this burden is refusing care, which is tantamount to abandoning the patient. That can be morally acceptable for people in exigent circumstances, but is generally difficult to justify, and for wealthy societies sets a dangerously unjust precedent" (Boyle, 1991, p. 17). This assumption leads to my third contention, that any financial burden at all upon the public purse to support the preservation of the lives of patients in PVS is extraordinary, and so not obligatory.

Before turning to the arguments supporting this contention, it is worthwhile to indicate the amount of monies involved. There are estimated to be between 15,000 and 25,000 persistently vegetative patients in the United States (Council on Scientific Affairs, 1990, p. 427). At a cost of $110,00 per patient per year, it would take between $1.65 billion and $2.25 billion to preserve their lives. The total cost of health care in the United States in 1989 was $604.1 billion, of which 33% or $199.7 billion was underwritten by private insurance and 41.9% or $253.3 billion by government programs (Levi et al., 1991, p. 123). Even if government paid for all of the costs of preserving the lives of permanently vegetative patients, the burden could not possibly be more than one percent of the total burden upon government for supporting health care. Those who think that the preservation of such life is morally obligatory, do not think that government support of it would be a significant burden upon taxpayers' resources. I argue to the contrary.

Even if those who must care for patients in PVS are obligated to tube feed them so long as the burden is not extraordinary, it does not follow that a secular pluralist society is so obligated. To show the obligation upon such a body politic, one must give cogent argument to show that the common good requires helping to underwrite the tube feeding of the permanently vegetative, or at least requires devoting those funds to this end rather than to other choiceworthy ends for which public funding is thought to be needed, e.g., education, the arts, housing, and helping to succor the lives of those who can (re)attain conscious function. Such an argument would not be needed if the citizens were explicitly to authorize funds for that end. But the fact that many citizens find such an end morally repugnant means that one needs good reason to authorize the government to coopt dissenting citizens' monies in order to pursue that end. My point is that even if there is moral obligation to tube feed patients in PVS, one needs additional argument to show that the state is morally authorized to impose that obligation upon its citizens. We get some argument in the form of a dilemma posed to those who, in an affluent society such as ours, would use financial costs to justify a decision not to feed the permanently vegetative:

Either food is withheld precisely as a means of saving the total cost of care or, at least, food is withheld as part of a more inclusive decision to save that total cost. If food is withheld precisely as a means of saving the total cost of care, the choice is to kill the comatose person, since the means achieves its end only by starving the person to death and rendering unnecessary any further care (except for disposal of the corpse). But ... the choice to kill the person would be homicidal and therefore, morally unjustifiable. If, however, food is withheld as part of a more inclusive decision to save the total cost of care, the issue no longer is whether comatose persons should be fed or not, but whether they should be cared for or abandoned. But the choice to abandon comatose persons bears on every element of their care, and so it cannot be justified by considerations which concern only either the technique by which they are fed or the appropriateness of medical treatment for persons in their situation. So, the real ... issue <is>: in our affluent society, can we justify abandoning the comatose in order to save the cost of caring for them as we care for others who cannot care for themselves? (Grisez, 1990, p. 35).

The argument is not cogent, however, because both horns of the dilemma can be avoided. With respect to the first, those who say that financial costs can relativize the duty to maintain life, do not thereby intend the death of patients; they would rejoice were a permanently vegetative patient miraculously to recover consciousness. If financial costs cannot relativize the duty to maintain life, then the distinction between ordinary and extraordinary means is invalid, as well as the rationale behind it, that life is ordained to higher, spiritual ends such that the means obligatory to maintain life should not render too difficult the attainment of those higher ends. With respect to the second horn, even if the costs were moderate and the monies at hand and not designated to other choiceworthy purposes, it is unclear that there is any duty to preserve the lives of patients in PVS. To employ medical resources to this end when the patients can neither benefit from these resources nor suffer from their withdrawal is arguably an inappropriate use of medical resources. To let such patients' lives expire in an appropriately dignified atmosphere is not to abandon them.

D. From a Secular Perspective. the Merely Biological Existence of a Patient In PVS Cannot Be Shown To Be the Existence of a Person

If *per impossible* one could restore such a patients to conscious function by modest expense, not to do so might seem closer to abandoning them than is the case in fact. Yet proponents of preserving their lives think that the life in a permanently vegetative state has the same moral worth as that of a human person, i.e., of a human capable of self-consciousness, reasoning about means and ends, and a moral sense developed enough to blame someone who gratuitously harms him. My fourth contention is that they are wrong.

The contention that humans incapable of exercising or developing any conscious function, e.g., patients in PVS, are nonetheless persons, is argued by means of a *reductio ad absurdum*.[11] If such a human were not a person, human life considered apart from any capacity for conscious function would be but the instrument of the reality that is capable of such function, i.e., of the person.[12] In this case, the argument goes, the life of the person and the person would be separable realities. This separability constitutes an indefensible dualism because it contradicts the starting point for thinking about the human person, viz., the reflective awareness of oneself as unitary. The human person cannot be separated from his manifestations in the world through his lived body; these manifestations must be ingredient in the unitary self of the human person. The person cannot be separated from the person's merely biological life. If PVS patients were once persons and still are living human beings, then they still are persons.

This argument, however, begs the question, namely, whether the human person is a separable reality from the merely biological life of its body, or an irreducibly distinct level of significance, one truly descriptive of a human being that can exercise the functions proper to a person, and not truly descriptive of a human being that cannot exercise these functions. If the person is a reality that is separable from its biologically living body, it has its own place, separate from the body's, in the causal sequences of events. To assert the protasis is in fact to assert an indefensible dualism, because the person's reality would then have to be, apart from any bodily manifestation, manifestable in a scientifically verifiable causal nexus. The sciences report no hint of transfer of energy due to a non-corporeal cause; quite the contrary, such a transfer would undermine the conservation of energy. If, on the other hand, the person is a distinctive significance of a human being who can manifest personal functions, its behavior cannot be adequately described in terms appropriate to a human being that cannot perform such functions; a person's characteristic behavior needs such terms as "praiseworthy" and "culpable" and "self-conscious" and "rational", i.e., personal predicates. There is, to be sure, a physiological correlate of such behavior: to be able to manifest such behavior, a human being must be able to have a functioning neocortex; the behavior of a human being without a functioning neocortex cannot be truly described by personal predicates. However, a physiologically adequate description of the behavior of human being with a functioning neocortex does not capture the significance of that behavior insofar as it is a person's; an additional level of description, one using personal predicates, is called for.[13] This view is not an indefensible dualism. It claims not that the human person is a reality separable from biologically human life, but that it is a significance that cannot be truly described of, cannot be present in, human life without a functioning neocortex. Life capable of manifesting behaviorially the functions of a person must be distinguished from human life without a neocortex and incapable of manifesting those functions.

It follows that, although merely biological human life is a necessary presupposition for being a person, its presence does not by itself entail the presence of a person. A human can have merely biological life and not be able to exercise any of the functions of a person. Patients in PVS do not have, and or incapable of having, functioning neocortexes. They are incapable of manifesting those behaviors that can only be adequately described in terms of personal predicates; they are incapable of exercising those functions that are necessary to mark a person. In terms of secular reason and experience, they do not have the status of persons.[14]

Consequently, their lives do not constitute the sort of good that is constituted by the lives of those who are (or, perhaps, can develop into) persons. In the lives of patients in PVS, there is no person present to respect. Such lives are incapable of self-consciousness; so they are incapable of recognizing as good any care that is given them. In contrast to infants and the severely mentally handicapped, they are not even capable of consciousness; so they can in no way appreciate care. Assume that one is obligated to do good to the particular humans which the rest of this paragraph discusses. One can then be said to have prima facie obligation to preserve the lives of human persons, even by invasive procedures (if the persons are not unwilling, and if the burden of putting the procedures into effect is not too great), because persons can value as good what is being done for them. But if human beings neither are nor can come to be persons, they cannot value anything, as good or otherwise. One still has a prima facie obligation to respect their bodily integrity: to provide them nourishment if it can be ingested naturally and is desired, to treat wounds such as cut arteries, and to provide comfort care where appropriate, i.e., where human beings may be capable of consciousness[15]; the consequences of not doing so would be drastic for one's regard of fellow human beings. In the case of patients in PVS, one is obligated to show the respect due to humans that once were persons, or at least are of a biological kind whose members are normally persons. (This respect would be manifested most obviously in hygienic care as the patients are allowed to expire.) However, there is no reason at all to preserve their lives invasively, except that it satisfies desires of their caretakers.

E. From a Christian Perspective One Is Obligated Not To Preserve the Lives of PVS Patients By Invasive Means

The distinction between the human person and the human being that is the basis for the previous paragraph is explicitly rejected in recent official Roman Catholic teaching about the status of human beings at the initial stages of their development (Congregation of the Doctrine of the Faith, 1987, p. 701; cf. Boyle, 1991, pp. 6–7). Nonetheless, my final contention is that from the perspective of orthodox Christianity one has the same sort of obligations towards humans as were outlined in the previous paragraph with one amplification: Toward the patient in PVS one not only has no obligation to preserve life by invasive means; one has, if anything, an obligation not thus to interfere with life as God has given it and allowed it transpire.

From the perspective of Christian faith, each human life has a non-instrumental value, i.e., is an intrinsic good, because God gives such value to men alone among His earthly creatures. Only within the context of faith is the value of a human life incapable of the functions of a person non-instrumental. Within this context each human life has irreplaceable value as it has been made by God, so that one is never obligated to prolong that life by invasive means if one is acting out of a respect for that life as God has made it. One can argue that it is licit invasively to prolong a human life if one thinks that something of value can be effected or appreciated by that human being in the course of the life thus prolonged. But patients in PVS cannot effect or appreciate any value. And since the value that others allege for artificially preserving the life of such patients has been found to be specious, it is difficult to know what of positive value could be effected by invasively preserving those lives.

Moreover, such a means of preserving those lives interferes with the very condition upon which we accept them as non-instrumentally valuable, the condition that each is thus made by God. If in the course of one's life one becomes permanently vegetative, just as if someone is born anencephalic, one's life is nonetheless non-instrumentally valuable because it fits God's plan. But part of every human life is its finitude. And if we interfere with its normal passage to death, we should have good reason thus to alter God's plan. There is none in invasively prolonging the life of a PVS patient, just as there is none in doing so for the anencephalic. From the standpoint of faith we know that the proper telos of every man is, in the words of the liturgy of the St. John Chrysostom, "a Christian ending to <one's> life, painless, blameless, peaceful; and a good defence before the dread Judgment Seat of Christ". One therefore properly cares for the patient in PVS by praying for that patient's Christian salvation rather than by artificially delaying, for no good reason, that life's normal passage to its telos. Thus to delay the normal coming to pass of God's plan is not only not obligatory but positively pernicious.[16]

III

A summary statement of what I hope to have accomplished in this paper may be helpful.

I first reviewed the ordinary-extraordinary distinction, the crucial point of which is that extraordinary means to preserve cannot be obligatory, because they are intemperate. That is to say, they would normally distract from attention that must be paid to other goods, e.g., of succoring a family or satisfying intellectual curiosity or enjoying art, or in a Christian context the most important good of all, attaining salvation.

184 THOMAS J. BOLE, III

I then argued five contentions. First, the lack of obvious benefit in tube feeding patients in PVS makes those bear the burden of proof who claim that tube feeding such patients is ordinary, in the sense of being obligatory. Second, these people must show that if one is obligated to care for a patient in PVS at all, one is obligated to preserve that patient's life by tube feeding rather than to insure that this life expires in dignity, viz., with hygienic care. Third, since proponents of the obligation to tube feed patients in PVS assume that it is morally legitimate to use tax monies to underwrite the costs of preserving the lives of such patients, they must, in addition to showing that there is a moral obligation tube feed these patients, also show that this moral obligation is the kind that the state ought to support by coopting the monies even of citizens who think it evil to prolong artificially such patients' lives. Fourth, in secular terms human life in a permanently vegetative state is not a good of the sort which, like human lives of those who are or can come to be persons, we seem to be prima facie obligated to preserve. Fifth, in Christian terms the good of human life in a permanently vegetative state is the sort of good that is violated if that life is preserved by invasive means rather than being allowed to expire. The upshot of my contentions is that the very distinction upon which those who claim that tube feeding is obligatory, viz., the distinction between ordinary means to preserve life and extraordinary means, suggests that their claim is false.[17]

NOTES

[1] The argument against considering merely biological human life, as in patients in PVS, to be something distinct from the life of the human person, is nicely expressed in Finnis *et al.* (1987, pp. 304–309).

[2] '[I]f [one is not ethically obligated to maintain a life that is not capable of reaching life's spiritual goals], then ... the lives of countless severely handicapped persons, including infants and the elderly, are regarded as worthless' (May, 1990, p. 86).

[3] The *Antwerp Extrordinisse Postijdinghe* of April 10, 1650, reported that '[t]hat in Sweden a fool had died who had claimed to be able to live as long as he wanted' (quoted in Lindeboom, 1978, p. 94). Surveying Descartes' writings about how to maintain his health, Lindeboom infers that Descartes thought 'the natural span of life to be more than a century' (1978, p. 96).

[4] Cronin (1958) gives an excellent overview of the history of this distinction. Bole (1990) gives a much briefer resume and shows its contemporary relevance.

[5] A standard example of this last is the revulsion felt by a virgin facing a physical examination by a coarse physician. Since the relevant burdens may oppress not only the patient but also the patient's family and/or caregivers, a more relevant example

today would be the revulsion often – and not unjustifiably – felt by healthcare workers in using so many resources to preserve artificially the lives of patients in PVS.

[6] Cf.: '[T]he notion of utility or proportionate hope of success and benefit as an essential part of our definition of ordinary means. Any means, therefore, that does not give definite hope of benefit is an extraordinary means' (Council on Scientific Affairs, 1990, p. 129).

[7] Cf. anecdotal evidence: 'This author has queried thousands of people across the country as to how many want artificial nutrition and hydration continued after a firm medical diagnosis of p.v.s., and no one has ever answered in the affirmative' (O'Rourke, 1989, p.192). The case of Helga Wanglie (*New York Times*, January 10, 1991, pp. A10, 13: county hospital in Minneapolis seeks court permission to turn off ventilator of patient in PVS that has private insurance and had earlier expressed the view that 'only He who gave life has the right to take life'; this paper's fifth contention, that the view attributed to Wanglie is compatible with ceasing tube feeding of patients in PVS, applies *a fortiori* to such patients that in addition need ventilator support) is notable because it is an exception to what O'Rourke found: *exceptio regulam probat*. Evidence that the Wanglie case does not disprove the rule, is the fact that several states with very strong right-to-life movements that had in the past effectively prevented legislatively endorsed health care proxies, e.g., New York and Massachusetts, have in the wake of the *Cruzan* decision passed proxy statutes.This fact suggests that there is strong public sentiment in behalf of felicitating legally recognized advanced directives limiting artificial means of preserving life.

[8] *Origins* 17:2 (January 21,1988), p. 547, on a case ultimately decided in favor of the patient's family asking for removal of artificial nutrition and hydration, *Gray v. Romeo and the State of Rhode Island*, United States District Court for the District of Rhode Island, Civil Action No. 870573B, October 17,1988.

[9] J. Bopp (1988) estimates that the actual costs of feeding a patient in PVS is $7.80 per day, or 2.6% of the total costs of artificially conserving the patient's life. This would make the total cost per year $109,500 in 1988 dollars, and of this just under $2850 would be required for feeding. Since the cost of medical inflation is rising at over 10% per annum, the cost in 1992 dollars can be conservatively estimated as in the body of the paper.

[10] Cf. Grisez (1990, p. 32), explaining why he has changed his mind and come to think that tube feeding patients in PVS is obligatory: 'I had assumed that feeding a comatose person by tube is in itself expensive. But I was not paying attention to the distinction between the cost of feeding such a person and the total cost of caring for him or her. Most of the cost is for other elements of care: providing a room with suitable furnishings and equipment, keeping it warm, having someone present to do *everything* that must be done (not only to provide food), and so forth. The food itself costs very little, and those who care for comatose persons spend only a small part of their time in feeding them'.

[11] Cf. Finnis *et al.*, 1987, p. 307): '[Although] there can be no strict demonstration of the thesis that human life is a basic good of the person ..., ... the thesis can be defended by.. a *reductio ad absurdum*. For the thesis that life is only an instrumental good necessarily presupposes a rationally indefensible conception of the human individual, namely, some kind of dualism'. A full discussion of the arguments

involved in the sentence here footnoted is provided by Wildes (1991).

[12] Cf. May (1990, p. 85): '[I]f we judge that someone's life is so burdensome that there is no longer any obligation to preserve it, are we not in essence saying that this person's life is no longer something good, but has now become a disvalue, a burden, and that, consequently, the person would be better off dead than alive?' Such a judgment 'denigrates the inherent value of human bodily life, regarding it as a good for the person, not of the person'.

[13] One may ask whether this additional significance just is the reality of the person, a spiritual reality, in the same sense as one may want to view the legal and political and economic structures of humans as real. My point, however, is that their peculiar reality is manifested not in their possession of material properties not found in the non-human world, but in an additional level of significance that does not accrue to things that are not shaped by persons. See Engelhardt (1973) for the theoretical foundations of this view.

[14] It is worth pointing out that this distinction between a human being that is a person and a human being that is not, i.e., between a human person and a human being, is not a distinction in the 'quality of life' of human beings, as if human life were a generic substrate to which are ascribed various qualitative attributes. Rather, as Aristotle observed with respect to the soul or principle of life (*De anima* II, 3, 414b20–34), the kind of life is fundamentally different in an entity capable of rational and spiritual functions than in one which is not: the former, whether human or not, would have to be accorded a dignity quite different from that implied by our comportment toward non-human animals not capable of such functions, e.g., porpoises and higher primates, which we can capture and use for entertainment and experiments.

[15] This is sufficient answer to May's concern (1990, p. 86) cited in note 2 above. It also indicates how I would answer two other concerns that arise with respect to one's obligations to patients in PVS, viz., that providing a patient with food and water is an ordinary and obligatory means to preserve his life if he can ingest it on his own, but extraordinary if it has to be administered, as is the case with any patient in PVS, by an invasive procedure; and that the cause of death in the case of such a patient from whom tube feeding is withdrawn or withheld is ultimately the fatal pathology of being unable to ingest food, not the withdrawing or withholding of the tube through which he can be invasively fed.

[16] I am indebted to Bishop Makarios for this point.

[17] This paper has significantly benefitted from comments by Bishop Vladika Makarios (Institute for Eastern Orthodox Studies, Houston) and Richard A. Wright (University of Oklahoma Health Sciences Center).

BIBLIOGRAPHY

Bole, T. J.: 1990, 'Intensive care units (ICUs), and ordinary means: Turning virtue into vice', *Linacre Quarterly* 57: 1 (February), 68–77.

Bopp, J.: 1988, 'Choosing death for Nancy Cruzan', *Hastings Center Report* 20: 1 (Jan–Feb), 38–41.

Boyle, J.: 1991, 'The Roman Catholic tradition and bioethics', in B. A. Lustig (ed.), *Bioethics Yearbook Volume I. Theological Developments, 1988–1990*, Kluwer

Academic Publishers, Dordrecht, pp. 5–20.

Congregation for the Declaration of the Faith: 1980, 'Declaration on euthanasia', reprinted in D. McCarthy and A. Moraczewsky (eds.), *Moral Responsibility in Prolonging Life Decisions*, Pope John XXIII Medical Moral Center, St. Louis, 1981.

Congregation for the Declaration of the Faith: 1987, 'Instruction on respect for human life in its origin and on the dignity of procreation' [also known as *Donum vitae*], *Origins* 16, 697–711.

Council on Scientific Affairs and Council on Ethical and Judicial Affairs: 1990, 'Persistent vegetative state and the decision to withdraw or withhold life support', *Journal of American Medical Association* 263: 3 (January 19), 426–430.

Cronin, D. A: 1958, *The Moral Law in Regard to the Ordinary and Extraordinary Means of Conserving Life*, Pontifical Gregorian University, Rome.

Engelhardt, H. T., Jr.: 1973, Mind-Body: *A Categorial Relation*, Martinus Nijhoff, The Hague.

Finnis, J., J. Boyle, and G. Grisez: 1987, *Nuclear Deterrence, Morality, and Realism*, Oxford University Press, Oxford.

Grisez, G.: 1990, 'Should nutrition and hydration be provided to permanently comatose and other mentally disabled persons?', *Linacre Quarterly* 57: 2 (May), 30–43.

Levit, K.R., H.C. Lazenby, S.W. Letsch, *et al.*: 1991, National health care spending, 1989', *Health Affairs* 10: 1, 117–130.

Lindeboom, G. A.: 1978, *Descartes and Medicine*, Rodopi, Amsterdam.

May, W. E.: 1990, 'Criteria for withholding or withdrawing treatment', *Linacre Quarterly* 57: 3 (August), 81–90.

Office of National Cost Estimates of the Health Care Financing Administration, 'National health expenditures, 1988', *Health Care Financing Review* 11: 4 (Summer 1990), 1–41.

O'Rourke, K.: 1989, 'Should nutrition and hydration be provided to permanently unconsciuos and other mentally disabled persons?', *Issues in Law and Medicine* 5:2, 183–196.

Pius XII, Pope: 1957, 'Le Dr. Bruno Haid' (address to the International Congress of Anesthesiologists, November 24, 1957), *Acta Apostolicae Sedis* 49, 1027–1033, this volume, pp. 209–215.

Wildes, K. W.: 1991, 'Life as a good and the obligations to persistently vegetative patients', in this volume, pp. 145–154.

JOHN J. PARIS S.J.

THE CATHOLIC TRADITION ON THE USE OF NUTRITION AND FLUIDS

In an important essay in the 1985 *Archives of Internal Medicine* entitled "Against the Emerging Stream", Siegler and Weisband note "that if five or even three years earlier anyone had seriously proposed removing food and water from a terminally or comatose patient, the very notion would have met strenuous objection". Yet, only five years after the publication of that article, the United States Supreme Court in *Cruzan v. Missouri State Hospital* ruled that a competent patient could refuse life-sustaining nutrition and fluids, and that, if evidentiary standards set by the state were met, a similar decision could be made for an incompetent patient. That shift in policy and practice precipitated a widespread and at times somewhat tumultuous debate on the morality of withdrawing nutrition and fluids from terminally ill, irreversibly comatose and severely demented patients, a debate in which moral theologians, and at times Catholic bishops, found themselves on opposite sides of the issue.

The debate began not as a speculative problem of moral theology, but in response to the indictment in 1983 of two California physicians for first degree murder for the removal, at the family's request, of an intravenous feeding line from an irreversibly comatose patient. The indictment was ultimately dismissed by the California Court of Appeals on the grounds that the physicians had no duty to provide an ineffective and futile medical intervention to a patient who had previously stated he would not want to be maintained in such a condition (*Barber v. Superior Court*).

A year later, the issue was raised again in a New Jersey Superior Court in the case of Claire Conroy, an eighty-four year old nursing home resident suffering from advanced dementia and irreversible physical arteriosclerotic heart disease, diabetes and hypertension. She could neither speak nor swallow and was fed by a nasogastric tube. She could smile or moan in response to stimuli, but was in a constricted semi-fetal position with no control over her bodily movements. Her nephew, who was her legal guardian, petitioned to have the nasogastric tube removed. Despite the testimony of the attending physician that the removal of the feeding tube would be an unacceptable medical practice, the trial judge

K.Wm. Wildes (ed.), Birth, Suffering and Death, 189–208.
© 1992 *Kluwer Academic Publishers. Printed in the Netherlands.*

authorized the removal because Miss Conroy's life had become intolerably and permanently burdensome.

Though Miss Conroy died while the decision was under appeal, the appellate division, believing the subject matter too important to be mooted by her death, reversed the trial court's judgment and stated that removal of the nasogastric tube would be tantamount to killing her *(Claire Conroy*, Appellate Division). A guardian's decision, the court argued, may never be used to withhold nourishment from an incompetent patient. In the court's words: "The trial judge authorized euthanasia [homicide]". In its view, "If the trial judge's order had been enforced, Conroy would not have died as the result of an existing medical condition, but rather she would have died, and painfully so, as the result of a new and independent condition: dehydration and starvation. Thus she would have been actually killed by independent means".

The New Jersey Supreme Court, the same court that had earlier issued the landmark *Quinlan* opinion (*Conroy*, 1985), reviewed the case and reversed the appellate division ruling. After acknowledging the right of a competent adult to decline medical treatment, it held that the right of a now incompetent patient such as Claire Conroy "remains intact even when she is no longer able to assert that right or to appreciate its effectuation" (*Conroy*, 1985). In elaborating on its reversal of the appellate division's judgment that cessation of artificial feeding was a homicide, the New Jersey Supreme Court asked: "In a case like that of Claire Conroy, for example, would a physician who discontinued nasogastric feeding be actively causing her death by removing her primary source of nutrients; or would he merely be omitting to continue the artificial form of treatment, thus passively allowing her medical condition, which includes her inability to swallow, to take its natural course?"

Its response was that artificial feeding by nasogastric tube or an intravenous line is equivalent to artificial breathing by a respirator, i.e., it is a medical procedure and as such should be provided or withheld on the same criteria as any other medical intervention: the proportionate burden and benefit to the patient. In the course of its analysis, the New Jersey Supreme Court cast aside several traditional distinctions as unhelpful: the distinction between actively hastening death and passively allowing it to occur; the distinction between withholding and withdrawing a treatment; the distinction between ordinary and extraordinary means.

This was particularly noteworthy both because these distinctions had been utilized by previous courts and by this court itself in *Quinlan*. An intervening factor, one the New Jersey Supreme Court utilized in its opinion, was the publication in 1983 of the report on *Deciding to Forgo Life-Sustaining Technologies* issued by the President's Commission for the Study of Ethical Problems in Medicine. That report, which borrowed liberally from traditional Catholic teaching on medical ethics, concluded that the language of the moralists on ordinary and extraordinary treatment had become so confused and misused that it was no longer useful. It urged that laws, judicial opinions, regulations, and medical policies speak instead, as did the Vatican's 1980 *Declaration of Euthanasia* (Sacred Congregation for Faith, 1980, pp. 154–157), of "proportionate benefits and burdens of treatment as viewed by particular patients". In doing so, the President's Commission was restoring the classical phrases to their original meaning.

In the decades prior to the 1983 California Court of Appeals' *Barber* opinion there had been virtually no discussion or analysis of withholding or withdrawing nutrition and fluids in the moral or medical literature. As a result, as Seigler's and Weisbard's article indicates, the practice had grown of routinely providing artificial nutrition and fluids to institutionalized patients unable to eat on their own.

Barber occasioned a burst of literature on the topic. An influential early article, one that actually predated *Barber*, was Joyce V. Zenwekh's "The dehydration question" in which a hospice nurse argued that it is not always more merciful to administer IV fluids to a dying patient. Rather, she believed we should examine the beneficial and detrimental effects of dehydration and then individualize the decision to the particular patient's condition and reaction to treatment.

Other articles soon followed from physicians and ethicists (Micetich, 1983; Childress and Lynn, 1983; Fletcher and Paris, 1983; Adlestein *et al.*, 1984) who argued that it is a medically and morally correct to omit IV fluids from dying or irreversibly comatose patients. The position was best summarized in James Childress and Joanne Lynn's essay "Must patients always be given food and water?" published in the 1983 *Hastings Center Report* in which they held that there are cases in which the best interest of the patient is served by omitting the provision of nutrition and fluids: when the procedure is futile, or if possible if no benefit to the patient (e.g., persistent vegetative state), or where the burden of edema, vomiting and mental confusion outweighs the benefits.This thesis found support even among traditional or conservative Catholic moralists. Albert S. Moraczewski, O.P. in an essay entitled "Is Food always obligatory?

Feeding the comatose patient" concluded "There appears to be no strict ethical obligation to provide nourishment by such technological interventions as intubation" (Moraczewski, 1985). And John Connery, S. J., criticized the New Jersey Supreme Court not for its ruling on the permissibility of withdrawing nutrition and fluids, but for its overly constricted interpretation of burden as limited to pain (Connery, 1985). In Connery's view, "the traditional moral approach was much broader. Besides pain, it would include other hardships " cost, or anything else the patient would consider burdensome".

Connery's conclusion on the morality of withdrawing nutrition and fluids from a patient in Ms. Conroy's condition is unambiguous: "From a moral perspective, we would judge that long-term use of a nasogastric tube might be very burdensome for a patient and therefore morally optional". As to the specifics of her case, he goes further than the court when he states, "If this was called for (and it seems to be the case), it would be morally permissible for Ms. Conroy (or her proxy following her wishes) to have the treatment withdrawn".

That seeming consensus among the Catholic commentators ended in 1986 when the New Jersey Catholic Conference, the organization of that state's Roman Catholic bishops, submitted an *amicus curiae* brief (New Jersey State Catholic Conference, 1987) to the New Jersey Supreme Court in the case of Nancy Jobes. The brief is remarkable in several ways. As Paul Armstrong, the attorney who represented the family of Karen Ann Quinlan and now represents the family of Nancy Jobes, observed: "It is hard to reconcile this brief with those submitted by the bishops earlier in the cases of Karen Ann Quinlan and Claire Conroy, and it is hard to reconcile the position advanced in Jobes with the longstanding teaching of the church" (Requena, 1986). The difficulty is that in the earlier cases, the bishops supported the termination of what was thought to be life-sustaining treatment for the irreversibly comatose Karen Quinlan and the removal of a feeding tube from the demented, dying Claire Conroy. Now the bishops are maintaining that "Catholic patients and their families, as well as caregivers, are obliged in all cases to accept, or to continue once begun, artificial medical measures that provide nutrition and hydration". Puzzled as well as troubled with the shift, Mr. Armstrong politely remarked, "I must say this latest statement is not my understanding of the fullest teaching of the Catholic Church".

Mr. Armstrong and the Catholic community are legitimately confused by the New Jersey bishops' recent statement. Examining the brief in more detail, reviewing the church's traditional teaching and pondering the reflections of moral theologians on the issue of withholding nutrition and fluids will help us uncover this confusion.

The bishops begin their statement by noting that: they are providing the court with "the moral and philosophical insights of Catholic ethical teaching" on the withholding of nutrition and fluids as it applies to the care of an individual such as Nancy Jobes (a Presbyterian being treated in a nonsectarian nursing home) and as it governs the practice of medicine in Catholic health-care facilities (Hill, 1986). They frame the issue, not in terms of the dignity of the individual, but as a concern for the right to life and society's duty to protect that right. They then forthrightly make their standard known: "Nutrition and hydration, which are basic to human life, and as such distinguished from medical treatment, should always be provided to the patient". Not to do so would, in their view, "introduce a new attack upon human life".

After admonishing the court not to draw its conclusion from an analysis of the "quality of life" of the patient, not to allow euthanasia and not to lessen the respect for the human life of the person who is seriously ill or dying, the bishops state that they "join the broad stream of ethical consciousness when we ask the court not to look favorably upon a plea sanctioning starvation as a means of death for a patient who would not otherwise die immediately". The bishops buttress their stand with a November 1985 statement from the Pontifical Academy of Sciences: "If the patient is in a permanent coma, irreversible as far as it is possible to predict, treatment is not required but *care, including feeding, must be provided*" (Pontifical Academy of Sciences, 1985). They also cite the Bishops' Committee for Pro-Life Activities (United States Bishops Committee, 1987) which states that since food and water can "generally be provided without the risks and burdens of more aggressive means of sustaining life, the law should establish a strong presumption in favor of their use".

The bishops conclude by urging the New Jersey Supreme Court to "stop the trend toward a public policy that does not advocate the preservation of life". Lest there be any doubt as to the "pro-life" stand they want protected, the bishops remind the court that "as long as evidence of human life is present, and it is present until death occurs, a living person exists". And that person, so long as he or she exists – regardless of condition, regardless of stated wishes, regardless of suffering and the burden of continued life – must be provided nutrition and fluids. To do otherwise, so the New Jersey bishops hold, would be intentional euthanasia. The New Jersey Supreme Court in its *Jobes* opinion passed over the bishops arguments in silence. It reiterated its earlier stand that nutrition and fluids were medical treatments that could be withheld or withdrawn based on the patient's physical condition and values.

Catholic leaders, though, did not remain silent on the issue. When the Council on Judicial and Ethical Affairs of the American Medical Association issued a statement at a New Orleans meeting on March 15, 1986, declaring that "life-prolonging medical treatment, including artificially or technologically supplied respiration, nutrition and hydration may be withheld from a patient in an irreversible coma even if death is not imminent" (AMA Judicial Council, 1988), New Orleans Archbishop Philip Hanna denounced the statement with the comment that:

The Catholic Church has always held that families are not obliged to use extraordinary means – such as artificial life support systems – to sustain the life of a patient in a hopelessly irreversible coma. However, food and water are ordinary means of sustaining life. Therefore, the Catholic Church opposes the American Medical Association's position because it approves denying a person the normal nourishment that he or she needs to sustain life (Hanna, 1986).

John Connery, who had earlier written in support of the removal of the nasogastric tube from Ms. Conroy, testified in the *Brophy* case against the removal of a gastrostomy tube from a forty-eight year old Massachusetts firefighter who failed to recover consciousness following neurosurgery for a massive cerebral aneurysm. Connery's arguments were incorporated in the trial judge's opinion which stated, "It is ethically inappropriate to cause the preventable death of Brophy by the deliberate denial of food and water that can be provided him in a noninvasive, nonintrusive manner that causes no pain and suffering, irrespective of the substitute judgment of the patient".

Connery elaborated on his arguments in an essay entitled "The Ethical Standards for Withholding/Withdrawing Nutrition and Hydration", (Connery, 1986). There, after indicating his belief that food and water are not medical treatments and that their removal from a patient must be aimed at bringing about death, Connery provides his major objection: Those who "would like to withhold or withdraw treatment on the basis of quality of life of the patient as well as the quality of means". His argument is that the assessment of the ordinary/extraordinary character of the treatment is to be made independently of the condition or subjective views of the patient. Since patients in a persistent vegetative condition such as Paul Brophy are no longer capable of experiencing pain or suffering, Connery concludes that it must be the diminished quality of their life that leads to the request to terminate treatment. For him the condition of the patient – or quality-of-his life – may not legitimately enter into the calculus.

Further, he believes quality-of-life judgments will inevitably prove to be a slippery slope, one that places large groups of vulnerable people at risk. In his words, "Today, we are intentionally ending the life of a person in an irreversible coma or persistent vegetative state. Tomorrow, it will be the person with Altzeimer's disease. The next day, any chronic mental patient will be considered. Then, or even before, incapacitating physical handicaps will be considered ... Eventually we will find ourselves in a society in which only those with an optimal quality of life will be secure".

Connery's concerns are not unique. Some one hundred physicians, moralists and others signed a document prepared by William E. May *et al.* on "Feeding and Hydrating the Permanently Unconscious and Other Vulnerable Persons" in which they argue that withholding or withdrawing food or fluids from those in a persistent vegetative state is euthanasia by omission. These patients are not terminally ill and so the action must be being done to end a life that is judged to be valueless or extensively burdensome. Such action is, they believe, "homicide". It is nothing other than a deliberate decision to kill these people by starvation and dehydration. May and colleagues, most of whom are theologians on Catholic faculties, understand the moral principle that "One may rightly choose to withhold or withdraw a means of preserving life if the means employed is judged either useless or excessively burdensome". And they correctly interpret the principle to mean that the technique is "too painful, too damaging to the patient's bodily self and functioning, too psychologically repugnant to the patient, too restrictive of the patient's liberty and preferred activities, too suppressive of the patient's mental life, or too expensive". But they restrict its application to patients who are imminently dying or those who cannot physically assimilate nourishment and fluids. That is, they insist the principle applies only when the use of the intervention would be futile or impossible. For patients such as Jobes or Brophy, who lie unresponsive in a persistent vegetative state, tube feeding is possible and, in their view, *not* useless. They argue "it produces great benefit, namely the preservation of their lives and the prevention of their deaths through malnutrition".

As to excessive burden to the family or community, factors which these commentators concede, have long been a consideration in Catholic moral theology, they contend that "the cost of providing food and fluids by entral tubes is not, in itself, excessive". The other care necessary to sustain the patient, care which in Paul Brophy's case cost $13,495 per month, they dismiss with the observation, "But these forms of care and maintenance are provided to many other classes of persons (e.g., those with severe mental illness or retardation, with long term disabilities, etc.)".

They do concede that harsh circumstances could render the provision of nutrition and fluids to the patient excessively burdensome, but conclude, "Our society is by no means in such straitened circumstances – in the *aftermath of nuclear destruction we may face such a situation*, but we are surely not facing one now" (Emphasis added).

One of those authors, Robert Barry, O. P., goes even further than the group. He would require "food and fluids be given to all patients until a certain determination of death has been made" (Barry, 1985). Lest his position be misunderstood, Barry explains, "Food and fluids should also be given to those who have been diagnosed as brain dead and who display other signs of vitality, for they are only in the final stages of dying, but are not yet dead". His proof that these patients are not dead: they maintain urine output. That demonstration of spontaneous integration of major organ systems is evidence enough for Barry that nutrition and hydration must be continued.

Kevin O'Rourke, O. P. would place the emphasis differently. Speaking of the goals of life, he states, "The most significant norm for determining whether life support should be utilized is that the spiritual goal of life is the ultimate criterion to measure whether means are proportionate or disproportionate" (O'Rourke, 1989). Following Pius XII's declaration that "Life, health, all temporal activities are in fact subordinated to spiritual ends" (Pius XII, 1958), O'Rourke holds that "When the potential for spiritual function is no longer present, then it seems that all treatment or care efforts which sustain physiological function are ineffective". Moreover, O'Rourke believes "when a therapy will make it more difficult to obtain one's spiritual goal, then it need not be utilized". O'Rourke's conclusion is that "If the cognitive affective potential is nonexistent, the person is still a human being, but a human being toward whom we do not have an ethical obligation to prolong life". If there is no benefit – physical or spiritual – to be gained from delaying death, O'Rourke would allow a fatal pathology to progress to its natural end.

Two Catholic bishops, Eugene A. Morino, former Archbishop of Atlanta, and Louis Gelineau, Bishop of Providence, Rhode Island, were asked to apply these norms to specific cases that were then before courts in their jurisdictions. In response to the 1989 request of Georgia's Fulton County Superior Court in the case of a quadriplegic man asking to turn off the ventilator keeping him alive, Archbishop Marino, citing the Vatican's 1980 *Declaration on Euthanasia*, concluded that the use of a ventilator was an "extraordinary means of preserving life" and so the patient was free to decide whether to continue its use, "even though such disruption will end in death" (Marino, 1988).

A year earlier, Bishop Gelineau had been asked by the lawyer for Marcia Gray, a Catholic who had been maintained in a persistent vegetative condition for two years, for an opinion on the moral legitimacy of removing the life-sustaining nutrition and fluids. Bishop Gelineau, acknowledging that the magisterium of the Church has not yet issued a definitive statement regarding the need to provide nutrition and hydration to the permanently unconscious person, noted that within the Church there are two theological opinions on the question: the first, that nutrition and hydration can be considered extraordinary means of sustaining life in certain circumstances; the second that fluid and nutritional support are always to be provided (Gelineau, 1988).

Bishop Gelineau assigned his moral theologian Father Robert McManus to review the case and to assist the family in reaching a conscientious decision in accord with Catholic moral theology. It was his opinion that

The medical treatments which are being provided the patient, even those which are supplying nutrition and hydration artificially, offer no reasonable hope of benefit to her. This lack of reasonable hope or benefit renders the artificially invasive medical treatments futile and thus extraordinary, and disproportionate and unduly burdensome. Moreover, the continuation of such medical treatments is causing a significant and precarious economic burden to Mrs. Gray's family.

It must be unambiguously clear that the primary intention of removing what has been competently judged to be extraordinary means of artificially prolonging the patient's natural life is to alleviate the burden and suffering of the patient and not to cause her death.

Bishop Gelineau, in an official statement, authorized the use of that opinion with the comment, "Father's opinion does not contradict

Catholic's moral theology and in no way supports or condones the practice of euthanasia".

Several months after Bishop Gelineau's intervention in the Rhode Island case, Bishop James McHugh of Camden, New Jersey, and a co-author of the William May statement, issued a position paper on nutrition and fluids that was to be taken as the official direction to be followed in his dioceses (McHugh, 1989). While acknowledging that more than one position is found among Catholic theologians on artificially assisted nutrition and fluids, he maintained that "discontinuing nutrition and hydration [in the unconscious but non-dying patient] does not simply allow the patient to die from some existing pathology, but introduces a new cause of death, that is, starvation and dehydration". From his perspective, nutrition and hydration should be continued in such patients. Further, he believes that its deliberate withdrawal is not morally justified.

Bishop McHugh concludes that respect for human life requires us to carefully study the implication of modern medical technology in the light of our Catholic moral heritage concerning the sanctity of life. Here he is echoing the Vatican Declaration's admonition that "Today it is very important to protect, at the moment of death, both the dignity of the human person and the Christian concept of life against a technological attitude that threatens to become an abuse". The Church does that by its understanding that life is a gift from God, a gift which we hold in trust, not a possession over which we have absolute dominion. It likewise recognized that death is a part of life; it is not the end of life but a transition on our pilgrimage into the fullness of eternal life with God. Hence neither man nor death is an absolute. Our duty to nourish, protect and preserve life as God's gift is a true, but limited, obligation.

What are the limits that our Catholic moral heritage have discerned as our obligation to preserve life? The Vatican Declaration puts it succinctly: "In the past moralists have replied that one is never obliged to use 'extraordinary' means". But as the Declaration makes clear, the confusion, misuse abuse of that term has rendered it less precise in our age and so it might be preferable and more accurate to speak of "proportionate" and "disproportionate" means.

In making that assessment, which the Vatican states belongs "to the conscience either of the sick person or those qualified to speak in the sick person's name", consideration must be made of "the type of treatment to be used, its degree of complexity or risk, its cost and the possibilities of using it, and comparing these elements with the results that can be expected, taking into account the state of the sick person and his or her physical and moral resources".

When the decision is made that the burden of the treatment outweighs the benefits to this specific patient given his or her medical condition and spiritual, financial and physical resources available to that patient, it is, in the Vatican's words, "permitted with the patient's consent to interrupt these means". "Such a refusal", says the Vatican, "is not the equivalent of suicide [or euthanasia]; on the contrary, it should be considered an acceptance of the human condition, or a wish to avoid the application of a medical procedure disproportionate to the results that can be expected, or a desire not to impose excessive expense on the family or the community". That being so, there is no need to undergo "forms of treatment that would only secure a precarious and burdensome prolongation of life so long as the normal care due to the sick person in similar cases is not interrupted".

The Vatican's *Declaration* is a summary of the centuries-long tradition of the Church on the duty to preserve life. Beginning with the teachings of Domingo Soto in the 16th century – that religious superiors could only require their subjects to use medicine that could be taken without too much difficulty through the Vatican's 1980 "Declaration on Euthanasia", there have been clear limits set on what one if obliged to undergo to preserve life. The most famous formula for that limitation was the distinction first proposed in 1595 by Domingo Banez (McCartney, 1980) between "extraordinary" and "ordinary" means, by which was meant measures proportionate to one's condition or state in life. Thus, if something were very costly or burdensome or if it did not offer substantial benefit to the patient, there was no moral obligation to use it. This standard applied even to life-saving measures.

That the doctrine has continued unchanged to the present day is seen in the Vatican's recent "Declaration on Euthanasia", which states: "It is permitted, with the patient's consent, to interrupt those means where the results fall short of expectation". Withdrawing treatment, in the Vatican's words, "is not the equivalent of suicide; on the contrary, it should be considered as an acceptance of the human condition, or a wish to avoid the application of a medical procedure disproportionate to the results that can be expected, or a desire not to impose excessive expenses on the family or community". That such treatments include even nourishment and fluid is seen in the recent policy on "The Rights of the Terminally Ill" (United States Bishops' Committee, 1987) issued by the Pro-Life

Committee of the U.S. Catholic Conference: "Laws dealing with medical treatment may have to take account of exceptional circumstances where even means of providing nourishment may be too ineffective or burdensome to be obligatory".

That statement, not the prefatory comments cited by the New Jersey Catholic Conference – that "nutrition and fluids can *generally* be provided without the risks and burdens of more aggressive means of sustaining life" – is the operative standard held and taught by the church. It recognizes that there are certain circumstances in which the patient's condition is so debilitated that any treatment would be futile or, if not futile, would prove so burdensome as to be nonobligatory. In those limited situations, the withholding of nutrition and hydration is designed not to hasten the death by starvation or dehydration, but to spare the patient the prolongation of life when the patient can derive no benefit from such prolongation.

The clearest statement of that teaching is found in the *Relationes Theologicae* by the 16th-century Dominican moralist Francisco DeVitoria (DeVitoria, 1587). In a commentary on the obligation to use food to preserve life, DeVitoria asks: "Would a sick person who does not eat because of some disgust for food be guilty of a sin equivalent to suicide?" His reply: "If the patient is so depressed or has lost his appetite so that it is only with the greatest effort that he can eat food, this right away ought to be reckoned as creating a kind of impossibility, and the patient is excused, at least from mortal sin, especially if there if little or no hope of life".

DeVitoria provides an everyday example of the type of "delicate treatment" that would be beyond what one is obliged to employ to preserve life: "Chickens and partridges, even if ordered by the doctor, need not be chosen over eggs and other common items, even if the individual knew for certain that he could live another 20 years by eating such special foods". If this was true of hens and partridges in DeVitoria's time, how much the more so today for total parenteral nutrition, feeding gastrostomies, nasogastric tubes and other artificial means of providing alimentation?

That DeVitoria's views were neither unique nor subsequently abandoned is best seen in a 1950 *Theological Studies* essay on "The Duty of Using Artificial Means of Preserving Life" by the widely respected Jesuit moralist Gerald Kelly. Kelly was concerned with the same questions now confronting the courts in O'Brien, Requena and Jobes: Is there a moral obligation to continue intravenous feeding of an irreversibly comatose, terminally ill patient? After a thorough survey of the prior teachings on the subject, Kelly finds that the authors hold that "no *remedy* is obligatory unless it offers a reasonable hope of checking or curing a disease (Nemo ad inutile tenetur)". From this Kelly concludes that no one is obliged to use any means – natural or artificial if it does not offer a reasonable hope of success in overcoming that person's condition.

Kelly's application of the principle is instructive. He immediately asks if all artificial means are remedies, or are some, such as intravenous feeding, merely designed to supplant a natural means of sustaining life? He quickly dismisses the speculative difference as irrelevant and insists that in the world of sick people, all artificial means of sustaining life are remedies for some diseased or defective condition. Kelly specifically applies this holding to the use of oxygen or intravenous feeding to sustain life in the so-called "hopeless" cases. His response is quite direct: "There is no obligation of using these things, unless they are needed to allow time for the reception of the sacraments". Practical application of principles is the mark of a moralist, and Kelly provides us with two cases – cases nearly identical to questions raised in the cases of Requena, O'Brien and Jobes. In his first example, a terminally ill cancer patient's painful death is being prolonged by intravenous feeding. With such therapy, the patient could survive several more weeks. The physician stops the intravenous feeding, and the patient dies soon thereafter. As is true in the present disputes, the commentators were divided over whether the intravenous feedings constituted an "ordinary" or "extraordinary" means of preserving life. Kelly concedes that one could consider the treatment as "ordinary". But one must still determine if the patient is obliged to undergo it. Kelly's answer is straightforward and clear: Since the prolonging of life is relatively useless, the patient may refuse the treatment. Further, he argues, if the patient is so racked with pain that he is unable to speak for himself, "the relatives and physicians may reasonably presume that he does not wish the intravenous feeding" and licitly discontinue it.

In the second case, Kelly goes even further. When asked if oxygen and intravenous feeding must be used to extend the life of a patient in a terminal coma, he replies: "I see no reason why even the most delicate professional standard should call for their use. In fact, it seems to me that, apart from very special circumstances, the artificial means not only need but should not be used, once the coma is reasonably diagnosed as terminal. Their use creates expense and nervous strain without conferring any real benefit".

A 1958 doctoral dissertation at the Gregorian University in Rome, "The Moral Law in Regard to the Ordinary and Extraordinary Means of Preserving Life", by Daniel A. Cronin (the present Archbishop of Hartford, Mass.) provides the most authoritative historical study of this topic. After a review of over 50 moral theologians, from Aquinas to those writing in the early 1950's, Cronin concludes that the church's teaching is consistent in its view: "Even natural means, such as taking of food and drink, can become optional if taking them requires great effort or if the hope of beneficial results (spes salutis) is not present". For the patient whose condition is incurable, Cronin writes, "even ordinary means, according to the *general norm*, have become extraordinary [morally dispensable] for the patient and [so] the wishes of the patient, expressed or reasonably interpreted, must be obeyed."

Cronin's retrospective analysis of the tradition firmly established that the moralists have always held that no means – including food or water – can be said to be absolutely obligatory regardless of the patient's status. How then did the idea that food and water must always be provided the patient gain currency? Perhaps it arose from the hesitancy expressed by Kelly to advise physicians that it is morally permissible to discontinue intravenous feeding lest such action be misinterpreted as a form of Catholic euthanasia.

That reluctance was intensified in Charles McFadden's widely circulated *Medical Ethics*, which was published in 1967. McFadden wrote that while the long-term use of artificial feedings could constitute a grave and nonobligatory burden, as a matter of practical medical advice he would never propose the removal of intravenous feeding once it had been instituted. The danger is that of scandal, guilt on the part of the family and misuse by insensitive or unscrupulous physicians. Those not familiar with nuanced distinctions, he argued, might believe that the patient had been deliberately killed to alleviate his suffering. Others then might all too readily terminate nourishment for anyone whose life was considered "useless". Opposition to the application of the traditional doctrine to medical practice soon led to the notion that what was theoretically correct was not only rash, it was wrong. From there it was an easy step to the position that it was wrong because it violated fundamental principles such as: "One must always use 'ordinary' means to preserve life".

The feeding issue fairly much dropped from the literature until the

Karen Ann Quinlan case once again brought it to public attention. Then Paul Ramsey, whose essay "On (Only) Caring for the Dying" has yet to be surpassed for insight and beauty in describing the Christian's responsibility toward the dying, adopted and updated Kelly's formulation. Ramsey's version reads: "Never abandon care". For the dying, Ramsey maintains that care is not recourse to pretended remedies; it is comfort and company. For those, such as Nancy Jobes, who are now beyond both, there is no objection to withholding or withdrawing nourishment. The application of the theory occurred when Ramsey equated the respirator and the intravenous treatment as equally aimless means of prolonging Karen Ann Quinlan's dying.

Ramsey's perspective was subsequently endorsed by Richard A. McCormick, S. J. (1982), when, during a June 1982 hearing at the President's Commission on Ethical Problems in Medicine, the question was asked whether there was any moral difference between removing a respirator, antibiotics or artificial feeding from Karen Ann Quinlan. The reply from the Catholic tradition was clearly, "No". If, for example, she were to contract pneumonia, there would be no need to use antibiotics because she would stand to gain nothing from such an intervention. A similar argument could likewise be made with regard to the continued use of feeding through the nasogastric tube. We were aware, as were McFadden and Kelly, of the danger of misinterpretation and misuse of the principle, and we were aware that there are forces in our society that would welcome the highly publicized withdrawal of nutrition from Quinlan as an invitation to active euthanasia. Hence we cautioned that it might be imprudent to withdraw the treatment in *her particular* well-publicized case.

Until such highly emotionally charged cased as Quinlan's, there was little ambiguity or hesitancy about ending artificial feeding for dying patients. For example, in his widely noted and frequently anthologized 1976 annual discourse to the Massachusetts Medical Society, "On Caring for the Patient With Cancer", Dr. J. Englebert Dunphy admonished physicians: "There is no need to prolong a useless and tragic life [of a patient racked with cancer] *by force feeding* or giving antibiotics ... to drag it out for a few more agonizing days or weeks". In his sharply stated summary: "That is the science without the humanity of medicine" (Dunphy, 1976).

And in an essay entitled "A Quiet Death, With Dignity" Cornelia Holbert (1977) wrote about her mother, an 86-year-old victim of multiple strokes whose newly contracted pneumonia was being treated by intravenous fluids and antibiotics. At her own request, the mother was disconnected from those (simple, ordinary and customary) treatments. She was kept comfortable by a fingertip dipped in ice water and smoothed over her tongue. During this time, her beloved rosary was placed in her hand. In Holbert's moving words, "Love flowed now, not merely love of compassion but the love of adoration for the glory of a soul stripped down to its pure white essence".

Holbert's essay evoked no charges of euthanasia; it conjured up no horrors of death by starvation and dehydration; it provoked no episcopal warnings of denigration of "life". Rather, it was received in simple story form as an exposition of the fervent Catholic prayer for the sick: "For speedy recovery or a happy death".

This understanding of life, death and the role of medicine continues to predominate in the thinking and writing of Catholic theologians. With the exception of Robert Barry, O. P., whose position parallels that of the New Jersey Conference's brief, it is not clear that there is any prominent theologian who maintains that nutrition and fluids must always be provided to all patients, including the terminally ill. For Barry that obligation persists even for those who are brain dead because, in his view, "They are only in the final states of dying, but not yet dead".

John Connery, S. J., testified against the removal of a feeding gastrostomy from 49-year-old Paul Brophy, an irreversibly comatose Massachusetts man, urging that we not fall into a "quality of life" standard. Nonetheless, Connery wrote of the demented, terminally ill Claire Conroy: "From a moral perspective we would judge that long-term use of a nasogastric tube might be very burdensome for a patient, and therefore morally optional". He continued: "If this was called for (and its seems to be the case), it would be morally permissible for Ms. Conroy (or her proxy following her wishes) to have the treatment withdrawn".

Two of Connery's theological colleagues at Chicago's Loyola University, David Thomasma (Micetich *et al.*, 1986), and James Walter (1986) have written in support of termination of life support. Thomasma, writing in *Critical Care Clinics*, argues that "certain circumstances make administration of food and water futile". In those situations, Thomasma believes, "To persist in indiscriminately using such gestures can convey stupidity and cruelty, not compassion and love". After reviewing the various positions offered in the Brophy case, Walter concluded, "I side with those who see no moral distinction between the refusal/withdrawal of various medical technologies". Similar positions have been taken by Varga, (Paris and Varga, 1984) and McCormick (1985), and by most of the Catholic moralists who have written on this topic including Dennis Brodeur, Albert Moraczewski, O.P., Gary Atkinson, Edward Bayer, James Bresnahan, S.J., David Thomasma, James Walters and Kevin O'Rourke, O.P.. That approach has likewise been taken in official guidelines on the use of nutrition and fluids in Catholic health care facilities by the Catholic Health Association of Wisconsin (1989) and the Roman Catholic Bishops of Texas (1990). The Wisconsin group declared that "Basic humane care must be maintained to make the patient's last days as comfortable as possible". That care includes oral nutrition and hydration but "medical techniques, including artificial nutrition and hydration can be withheld or withdrawn if the treatments are ineffective or burdensome for the patient". The guidelines conclude, "The fact that death occurs from the disease process after one withholds or withdraws ineffective or burdensome treatment is not euthanasia or suicide".

The Texas bishops outline the reasoning in the Vatican's *Declaration* and then apply it to the patient in a persistent vegetative state. Their analysis of such patients differs substantially from those who would describe them as "unconscious but non-dying". The Texas bishops describe the PVS patient as "human beings" who "are stricken with a lethal pathology which, without artificial nutrition and hydration, will lead to death". If there is evidence the now irreversibly comatose patient would not want to be maintained by artificial nutrition and fluids, these may be foregone or withdrawn. Such an action, in the bishops' understanding, "is not abandoning the person. Rather, it is accepting the fact that the person has come to the end of his or her pilgrimage and should not be impeded from taking the final step".

This subordination of physiological concerns to the patient's spiritual needs and obligations is the hallmark of authentic Catholic thinking. It is based on a clear and careful reiteration of the ethical assumptions upon which medicine and the efforts to treat people have been based – "to prolong living in order to pursue the purpose of life". The burden a person would experience in striving to obtain the purpose of life – not the burden associated with the means to prolong it – is and traditionally has been the focus of Catholic moral concern.

Then, it is this bedrock teaching of theology on the meaning of life and death – neither of which in the Christian framework ought to be made absolute – and not a misplaced debate on "the casuistry of means" that should guide our judgments on the difficult and sometimes trying decisions cast up by modern medical technology. To do otherwise – or to count mere vegetative existence as a patient-benefit – is to let slip one's grasp on the heart of Catholic tradition in this matter. It is that tradition, developed over centuries of living out the Gospel message on the meaning of life and death – and not some immediate political "pro-life" agenda – that is and ought to be the source of the Catholic Church's teaching on the use of nutrition and fluids.

BIBLIOGRAPHY

Adlestein, S. J., R. E. Cranford, S. H. Wanzer, *et al.*: 1984, 'The physician's responsibility toward the hopelessly ill patient', *The New England Journal of Medicine* 310, 955–959.

AMA Judicial Council: 1988, *Current Opinions of the Judicial Council of the American Medical Association*, American Medical Association, Chicago.

Archbishop Eugene A. Marino: 1988, 'Brief by Atlanta Archdiocese *In re Larry James McAfee*', Origins 19, 274–279.

Archbishop Phillip Hanna's: 1986 'Feeding the comatose and the common good in the Catholic tradition', P. Barry *The Thomist* 53, pp. 1–30.

Barry, R. L.: 1985, 'The ethics of providing life-sustaining nutrition and fluids to incompetent patients', *The Journal of Family and Culture* 1, 23–37.

Barry, R., O. Griese, W. E. May, *et al.*: 1987, 'Feeding and hydrating the permanently unconscious and other vulnerable, persons', *Issues in Law & Medicine* 3, 203–217.

Bishop James McHugh: October 12, 1989, 'Principles in, regard to withholding or withdrawing artificially assisted nutrition/hydration', *Origins*, 314–316.

Bishop Louis Gelineau: 1988, 'Brief on *In re Maria Gray*', *Origins* 21, 546–547.

Bishops of Texas and Texas Conference of Catholic Health Facilities: June 7, 1990, 'An interim pastoral statement on artificial nutrition and hydration', *Origins* 20, N.4.

Catholic Health Association of Wisconsin: 1989, 'Nutrition and Hydration Guidelines'.

Childress, J. F. and Lynn, J.: October 1983, 'Must patients always be given food and water?' *Hastings Center Report* 13, 17–21.

Connery, J. R.: 1986, 'The ethical standards for withholding/withdrawing nutrition and Hydration', *Issues in Law & Medicine* 2, 87–97.

Connery, J. R.: 1985, 'In the matter of Claire Conroy', *Linacre Quarterly* 52, 321–328.

Cronin, D. A.: 1958, *The Moral Law In Report to the Ordinary and Extraordinary Means of Conserving Life* (Dissertatio ad Laudem in Facultate Theologica Pontificae Universitatis Gregorianae), Romae.

DeVitoria, F.: 1587, 'Relectio de Temperentia', *Reflectiones Theologicae*, Lugdundi.

Dunphy, J. E.: 1976, 'On caring for the patient with cancer', *The New England Journal of Medicine* 295, 313–319.

Fletcher, A. B. and Paris, J. J.: 1983, 'Infant doe regulations and the absolute requirement to use nourishment and fluids for the dying infant', *Law, Medicine & Health Care*, 210–213.

Hill, P. T.: 1986, 'Defining sacred bonds: A lawyer looks at church, law & medical policy', *Commonweal* 113, 620–622.

Holbert, C.: 1977, 'A quiet death with dignity', *America* 136, 214–216.

Kelly, G.: 1950, 'The duty of using artificial means of preserving life', *Theological Studies* 12, 550–556.

McCartney, J. J.: 1980, 'The development of the doctrine of ordinary and extraordinary means of preserving life in catholic moral theology before the Karen Quinlan Case', *Linacre Quarterly* 47, 215–226.

McCormick, R. A.: 6, 1985, 'Caring or starving? The case of Claire Conroy', *America* 152, 269–273.

McCormick, R. A.: 1982, 'Transcript of proceedings, President's Commission for the Study of Ethical Problems in Medicine and Biomedical and Behavioral Research', Meeting No. 21, p. 98.

McFadden, C. J.: 1967, *Medical Ethics*, F.A. Davis Co., Philadelphia, Pennsylvania.

Micetich, K., P. H. Steinecker, D. Thomasma: 1986, 'Continuance of nutritional care in the terminally ill patient', *Critical Care Clinics* 2, 61–71.

Micetich, K., P. H. Steinecker, D. Thomasma: 1983, 'Are intravenous fluids morally required for a dying patient?– *Archives of Internal Medicine* 143, 975–978.

Moraczewski, A. S.: 1985, 'Is food always obligatory? Feeding the comatose patient', *Ethics & Medicine* 10, 13–4, 9.

New Jersey State Catholic Conference Brief: 1987, 'Providing food and fluids to severely brain damaged Patients', *Origins* 16, 582–584.

O'Rourke, K.: 1989, 'Should nutrition and hydration be provided to permanently unconscious and other mentally disabled persons?', *Issues in Law & Medicine* 5, 181–196.

Paris, J. J. and McCormick, R. A.: 'The catholic tradition on the use of nutrition and fluids', *America*, May 2, 1987, pp. 356–361.

Paris, J. J., and Varga, A. C.: 1984, 'Care of the Hopelessly Ill', *America* 151, 141–144.Pius XII: 1958, 'The Prolongation of Life', *Pope Speaks* 4, 393–398.

President's Commission for the Study of Ethical Problems in Medicine and Biomedical and Behavioral Research: 1983, *Deciding to Forego Life-Sustaining Treatment*, U. S. Government Printing Office, Washington, D. C.

Ramsey, P.: 1970, 'On (only) caring for the dying', *The Patient as Person*, Yale University Press, New Haven, Connecticut.

Sacred Congregation for Faith: 1980, 'Declaration on Euthanasia', *Origins* 10, 154–157.

Siegler, M. and Weisband A.: 1985, 'Against the emerging stream: Should fluids and nutritional support be discontinued?', *Archives of Internal Medicine* 145, 129–131.

Statement of the Pontifical Academy of Sciences: 1985, *L'Osservatore Romano*, 10.

United States Bishops' Committee for Pro-Life Activities: 1987, The rights of the terminally ill', *Origins* 16, 222–226.

Walter, J. J.: 1986, 'Food and water: An ethical burden: The withdrawal of artificial nutrition', *Commonweal* 113, 616–619, at 619.

Zerwekh, Joyce: 1983, 'The dehydration question', *Nursing*, 47–51.

CASES AND STATUTES

Barber v. Superior Court, 147 Cal. App.3rd 1006, 195 Cal. Rptr. 484 (1983).
Brophy v. New England Sinai Hospital, No.85E0009–G1, Mass. Probate and Family Court, Norfolk, MA. (October 21, 1985).
Cruzan v. Director, Missouri Department of Health, 110 S.Ct. 2841 (1990).
In re Conroy, 98 N. J. 321, 486 A.2d 1209 (1985).
In re Quinlan, 70 N. J. 10, 355 A.2d 647 (1985).
In re Nancy Jobes, 108 N. J. 394, 529 A.2d 434 (1987).
In re Requena, No.P–326–86E (Ch. Div. Sept. 24, 1986), aff'N. J. Super. (App. Div. 1986).

POPE PIUS XII

THE PROLONGATION OF LIFE

Dr. Bruno Haid, chief of the anesthesia section at the surgery clinic of the University of Innsbruck, has submitted to Us three questions on medical morals treating the subject known as "resuscitation" [*la réanimation*].

We are pleased, gentlemen, to grant this request, which shows your great awareness of professional duties, and your will to solve in the light of the principles of the Gospel the delicate problems that confront you.

PROBLEMS OF ANESTHESIOLOGY

According to Dr. Haid's statement, modern anesthesiology deals not only with problems of analgesia and anesthesia properly so-called, but also with those of "resuscitation." This is the name given in medicine, and especially in anesthesiology, to the technique which makes possible the remedying of certain occurrences, which seriously threaten human life, especially asphyxia, which formerly, when modern anesthetizing equipment was not yet available, would stop the heart and bring about death in a few minutes. The task of the anesthesiologist has therefore extended to acute respiratory difficulties, provoked by strangulation or by open wounds of the chest. The anesthesiologist intervenes to prevent asphyxia resulting from the internal obstruction of breathing passages by the contents of the stomach or by drowning, to remedy total or partial respiratory paralysis in cases of serious tetanus, of poliomyelitis, of poisoning by gas, sedatives, or alcoholic intoxication, or even in cases of paralysis of the central respiratory apparatus caused by serious trauma of the brain.

THE PRACTICE OF "RESUSCITATION"

In the practice of resuscitation and in the treatment of persons who have suffered headwounds, and sometimes in the case of persons who have undergone brain surgery or of those who have suffered trauma of the brain through anoxia and remain in a state of deep unconsciousness, there

K.Wm. Wildes (ed.), Birth, Suffering and Death, 209–215.
© 1992 *Kluwer Academic Publishers. Printed in the Netherlands.*

arise a number of questions that concern medical morality and involve the principles of the philosophy of nature even more than those of analgesia.

It happens at times – as in the aforementioned cases of accidents and illnesses, the treatment of which offers reasonable hope of success – that the anesthesiologist can improve the general condition of patients who suffer from a serious lesion of the brain and whose situation at first might seem desperate. He restores breathing either through manual intervention or with the help of special instruments, clears the breathing passages, and provides for the artificial feeding of the patient.

Thanks to this treatment, and especially through the administration of oxygen by means of artificial respiration, a failing blood circulation picks up again and the appearance of the patient improves, sometimes very quickly, to such an extent that the anesthesiologist himself, or any other doctor who, trusting his experience, would have given up all hope, maintains a slight hope that spontaneous breathing will be restored. The family usually considers this improvement an astonishing result and is grateful to the doctor.

If the lesion of the brain is so serious that the patient will very probably, and even most certainly, not survive, the anesthesiologist is then led to ask himself the distressing question as to the value and meaning of the resuscitation processes. As an immediate measure he will apply artificial respiration by intubation and by aspiration of the respiratory tract: he is then in a safer position and has more time to decide what further must be done. But he can find himself in a delicate position, if the family considers that the efforts he has taken are improper and opposes them. In most cases this situation arises, not at the beginning of resuscitation attempts, but when the patient's condition, after a slight improvement at first, remains stationary and it becomes clear that only automatic artificial respiration is keeping him alive. The question then arises if one must, or if one can, continue the resuscitation process despite the fact that the soul may already have left the body.

The solution to this problem, already difficult in itself, becomes even more difficult when the family – themselves Catholic perhaps – insists that the doctor in charge, especially the anesthesiologist, remove the artificial respiration apparatus in order to allow the patient, who is already virtually dead, to pass away in peace.

A FUNDAMENTAL PROBLEM

Out of this situation there arises a question that is fundamental from the point of view of religion and the philosophy of nature. When, according to Christian faith, has death occurred in patients on whom modern methods of resuscitation have been used? Is Extreme Unction valid, at least as long as one can perceive heartbeats, even if the vital functions properly so-called have already disappeared, and if life depends only on the functioning of the artificial-respiration apparatus?

THREE QUESTIONS

The problems that arise in the modern practice of resuscitation can therefore be formulated in three questions:

First, does one have the right, or is one even under the obligation, to use modern artificial-respiration equipment in all cases, even those which, in the doctor's judgment, are completely hopeless?

Second, does one have the right, or is one under obligation, to remove the artificial-respiration apparatus when, after several days, the state of deep unconsciousness does not improve if, when it is removed, blood circulation will stop within a few minutes? What must be done in this case if the family of the patient, who has already received the last sacraments, urges the doctor to remove the apparatus? Is Extreme Unction still valid at this time?

Third, must a patient plunged into unconsciousness through central paralysis, but whose life – that is to say, blood circulation – is maintained through artificial respiration, and in whom there is no improvement after several days, be considered "*de facto*" or even "*de jure*" dead? Must one not wait for blood circulation to stop, in spite of the artificial respiration, before considering him dead?

BASIC PRINCIPLES

We shall willingly answer these three questions. But before examining them We would like to set forth the principles that will allow formulation of the answer.

Natural reason and Christian morals say that man (and whoever is entrusted with the task of taking care of his fellowman) has the right and the duty in case of serious illness to take the necessary treatment for the preservation of life and health. This duty that one has toward himself, toward God, toward the human community, and in most cases toward certain determined persons, derives from well ordered charity, from submission to the Creator, from social justice and even from strict justice, as well as from devotion toward one's family.

But normally one is held to use only ordinary means – according to circumstances of persons, places, times and culture – that is to say, means that do not involve any grave burden for oneself or another. A more strict obligation would be too burdensome for most men and would render the attainment of the higher, more important good too difficult. Life, health, all temporal activities are in fact subordinated to spiritual ends. On the other hand, one is not forbidden to take more than the strictly necessary steps to preserve life and health, as long as he does not fail in some more serious duty.

ADMINISTRATION OF THE SACRAMENTS

When the administration of sacraments to an unconscious man is concerned, the answer is drawn from the doctrine and practice of the Church which, for its part, follows the Lord's will as its rule of action. Sacraments are meant, by virtue of divine institution, for men of this world who are in the course of their earthly life, and, except for baptism itself, presuppose prior baptism of the recipient. He who is not a man, who is not yet a man, or is no longer a man, cannot receive the sacraments. Furthermore, if someone expresses his refusal, the sacraments cannot be administered to him against his will. God compels no one to accept sacramental grace.

When it is not known whether a person fulfills the necessary conditions for valid reception of the sacraments, an effort must be made to solve the doubt. If this effort fails, the sacrament will be conferred under at least a tacit condition (with the phrase "*Si capas est,*" "If you are capable," – which is the broadest condition). Sacraments are instituted by Christ for men in order to save their souls. Therefore, in cases of extreme necessity, the Church tries extreme solutions in order to give man sacramental grace and assistance.

THE FACT OF DEATH

The question of the fact of death and that of verifying the fact itself ("*de factor*") or its legal authenticity ("*de jure*") have, because of their consequences, even in the field of morals and of religion, an even greater importance. What We have just said about the presupposed essential elements for the valid reception of a sacrament has shown this. But the importance of the question extends also to effects in matters of inheritance, marriage and matrimonial processes, benefices (vacancy of a benefice), and to many other questions of private and social life.

It remains for the doctor, and especially the anesthesiologist, to give a clear and precise definition of "death" and the "moment of death" of a patient who passes away in a state of unconsciousness. Here one can accept the usual concept of complete and final separation of the soul from the body; but in practice one must take into account the lack of precision of the terms "body" and "separation." One can put aside the possibility of a person being buried alive, for removal of the artificial respiration apparatus must necessarily bring about stoppage of blood circulation and therefore death within a few minutes.

In case of insoluble doubt, one can resort to presumptions of law and of fact. In general, it will be necessary to presume that life remains, because there is involved here a fundamental right received from the Creator, and it is necessary to prove with certainty that it has been lost.

We shall now pass to the solution of the particular questions.

A DOCTOR'S RIGHTS AND DUTIES

1. Does the anesthesiologist have the right, or is he bound, in all cases of deep unconsciousness, even in those that are considered to be completely hopeless in the opinion of the competent doctor, to use modern artificial respiration apparatus even against the will of the family?

In ordinary cases one will grant that the anesthesiologist has the right to act in this matter, but he is not bound to do so, unless this becomes the only way of fulfilling another certain moral duty.

The rights and duties of the doctor are correlative to those of the patient. The doctor, in fact, has no separate or independent right where the patient is concerned. In general he can take action only if the patient explicitly or implicitly, directly or indirectly, gives him permission. The technique of resuscitation which concerns us here does not contain anything immoral in itself. Therefore the patient, if he were capable of making a personal decision, could lawfully use it and, consequently, give the doctor permission to use it. On the other hand, since these forms of treatment go beyond the ordinary means to which one is bound, it cannot be held that there is an obligation to use them nor, consequently, that one is bound to give the doctor permission to use them.

The rights and duties of the family depend in general upon the presumed will of the unconscious patient if he is of age and "*sui juris.*" Where the proper and independent duty of the family is concerned, they are usually bound only to the use of ordinary means.

Consequently, if it appears that the attempt at resuscitation constitutes in reality such a burden for the family that one cannot in all conscience impose it upon them, they can lawfully insist that the doctor should discontinue these attempts, and the doctor can lawfully comply. There is not involved here a case of direct disposal of the life of the patient, nor of euthanasia in any way: this would never be licit. Even when it causes the arrest of circulation, the interruption of attempts at resuscitation is never more than an indirect cause of the cessation of life, and one must apply in this case the principle of double effect and of "*voluntarium in causa.*"

EXTREME UNCTION

2. We have, therefore, already answered the second question in essence: "Can the doctor remove the artificial respiration apparatus before the blood circulation has come to a complete stop? Can he do this, at least, when the patient has already received Extreme Unction? Is this Extreme Unction valid when it is administered at the moment when circulation ceases, or even after?"

We must give an affirmative answer to the first part of this question, as We have already explained. If Extreme Unction has not yet been administered, one must seek to prolong respiration until this has been done. But as far as concerns the validity of Extreme Unction at the moment when blood circulation stops completely or even after this moment, it is impossible to answer "yes" or "no."

If, as in the opinion of doctors, this complete cessation or circulation means a sure separation of the soul from the body, even if particular organs go on functioning, Extreme Unction would certainly not be valid, for the recipient would certainly not be a man anymore. And this is an indispensable condition for the reception of the sacraments.

If, on the other hand, doctors are of the opinion that the separation of the soul from the body is doubtful, and that this doubt cannot be solved, the validity of Extreme Unction is also doubtful. But, applying her usual rules: "The sacraments are for men" and "In case of extreme necessity one tries extreme measures," the Church allows the sacrament to be administered conditionally in respect to the sacramental sign.

WHEN IS ONE "DEAD"?

3. "When the blood circulation and the life of a patient who is deeply unconscious because of a central paralysis are maintained only through artificial respiration, and no improvement is noted after a few days, at what time does the Catholic Church consider the patient 'dead,' or when must he be declared dead according to natural law (questions '*de facto*' and '*de jure*')?"

(Has death already occurred after grave trauma of the brain, which has provoked deep unconsciousness and central breathing paralysis, the fatal consequences of which have nevertheless been retarded by artificial respiration? Or does it occur, according to the present opinion of doctors, only when there is complete arrest of circulation despite prolonged artificial respiration?)

Where the verification of the fact in particular cases is concerned, the answer cannot be deducted from any religious and moral principle and, under this aspect, does not fall within the competence of the Church. Until an answer can be given, the question must remain open. But considerations of a general nature allow us to believe that human life continues for as long as its vital functions – distinguished form the simple life or organs – manifest themselves spontaneously or even with the help of artificial processes. A great number of these cases are the object of insoluble doubt, and must be dealt with according to the presumptions of law and of fact of which We have spoken.

May these explanations guide you and enlighten you when you must solve delicate questions arising in the practice of your profession. As a token of divine favors which We call upon you and all of those who are dear to you. We heartily grant you Our Apostolic Blessing.

Reprinted with permission of the editors from *The Pope Speaks*, vol. 4, 1958.

SACRED CONGREGATION FOR THE DOCTRINE OF THE FAITH

DECLARATION ON EUTHANASIA

INTRODUCTION

The rights and values pertaining to the human person occupy an important place among the questions discussed today. In this regard, the Second Vatican Ecumenical Council solemnly reaffirmed the lofty dignity of the human person, and in a special way his or her right to life. The Council therefore condemned crimes against life "such as any type of murder, genocide, abortion, euthanasia, or willful suicide" (Pastoral Constitution *Gaudium et spes*, no. 27).

More recently, the Sacred Congregation for the Doctrine of the Faith has reminded all the faithful of Catholic teaching on procured abortion.[1] The Congregation now considers it opportune to set forth the Church's teaching on euthanasia.

It is indeed true that, in this sphere of teaching, the recent Popes[2] have explained the principles, and these retain their full force; but the progress of medical science in recent years has brought to the fore new aspects of the question of euthanasia and these aspects call for further elucidation on the ethical level.

In modern society, in which even the fundamental values of human life are often called into question, cultural change exercises an influence upon the way of looking at suffering and death; moreover, medicine has increased its capacity to cure and to prolong life in particular circumstances, which sometimes gives rise to moral problems. Thus people living in this situation experience no little anxiety about the meaning of advanced old age and death. They also begin to wonder whether they have the right to obtain for themselves or their fellowmen an "easy death," which would shorten suffering and which seems to them more in harmony with human dignity.

A number of Episcopal Conferences have raised questions on this subject with the Sacred Congregation for the Doctrine of the Faith. The Congregation, having sought the opinion of experts on the various aspects of euthanasia, now wishes to respond to the Bishops' questions with the

K.Wm. Wildes (ed.), Birth, Suffering and Death, 217–224.
© 1992 *Kluwer Academic Publishers. Printed in the Netherlands.*

present Declaration, in order to help them to give correct teaching to the faithful entrusted to their care, and to offer them elements for reflection that they can present to the civil authorities with regard to this very serious matter.

The considerations set forth in the present document concern in the first place all those who place their faith and hope in Christ, who, through His life, death and resurrection, has given a new meaning to existence and especially to the death of the Christian, as St. Paul says: "If we live, we live to the Lord, and if we die, we die to the Lord" (Rom. 14: 8; cd. Phil. 1: 20).

As for those who profess other religions, many will agree with us that faith in God the Creator, Provider and lord of life – if they share this belief – confers a lofty dignity upon every human person and guarantees respect for him or her.

It is hoped that this Declaration will meet with the approval of many people of good will, who, philosophical or ideological differences notwithstanding, have nevertheless a lively awareness of the rights of the human person. These rights have often, in fact, been proclaimed in recent years through declarations issued by International Congresses[3]; and since it is a question here of fundamental rights inherent in every human person, it is obviously wrong to have recourse to arguments from political pluralism or religious freedom in order to deny the universal value of those rights.

I. THE VALUE OF HUMAN LIFE

Human life is the basis of all goods, and is the necessary source and condition of every human activity and of all society. Most people regard life as something sacred and hold that no one may dispose of it at will, but believers see in life something greater, namely, a gift of God's love, which they are called upon to preserve and make fruitful. And it is this latter consideration that gives rise to the following consequences:

1. No one can make an attempt on the life of an innocent person without opposing God's love for that person, without violating a fundamental right, and therefore without committing a crime of the utmost gravity.[4]

2. Everyone has the duty to lead his or her life in accordance with God's plan. That life is entrusted to the individual as a good that must bear fruit already here on earth, but that finds it full perfection

only in eternal life.

3. Intentionally causing one's own death, or suicide, is therefore equally as wrong as murder; such an action on the part of a person is to be considered as a rejection of God's sovereignty and loving plan. Furthermore, suicide is also often a refusal of love for self, the denial of the natural instinct to live, a flight from the duties of justice and charity owed to one's neighbor, to various communities or to the whole of society although, as is generally recognized, at times there are psychological factors present that can diminish responsibility or even completely remove it.

However, one must clearly distinguish suicide from that sacrifice of one's life whereby for a higher cause, such as God's glory, the salvation of souls or the service of one's brethren, a person offers his or her own life or puts it in danger (cf. Jn. 15: 14).

II. EUTHANASIA

In order that the question of euthanasia can be properly dealt with, it is first necessary to define the works used.

Etymologically speaking, in ancient times *euthanasia* meant an *easy death* without severe suffering. Today one no longer thinks of this original meaning of the word, but rather of some intervention of medicine whereby the suffering of sickness or of the final agony are reduced, sometimes also with the danger of suppressing life prematurely. Ultimately, the word *euthanasia* is used in a more particular sense to mean "mercy killing," for the purpose of putting an end to extreme suffering, or saving abnormal babies, the mentally ill or the incurably sick from the prolongation, perhaps for many years, of a miserable life, which could impose too heavy a burden on their families or on society.

It is, therefore, necessary to state clearly in what sense the word is used in the present document.

By euthanasia is understood an action or an omission which of itself or by intention causes death, in order that all suffering may in this way be eliminated. Euthanasia's terms of reference, therefore, are to be found in the intention of the will and in the methods used.

It is necessary to state firmly once more that nothing and no one can in any way permit the killing of an innocent human being, whether a fetus or an embryo, an infant or an adult, an old person, or one suffering from an incurable disease, or a person who is dying. Furthermore, no one is permitted to ask for this act of killing, either for himself or herself or for another person entrusted to his or her care, nor can he or she consent to it, either explicitly or implicitly. Nor can any authority legitimately recommend or permit such an action. For it is a question of the violation of the divine law, an offense against the dignity of the human person, a crime against life, and an attack on humanity.

It may happen that, by reason of prolonged and barely tolerable pain, for deeply personal or other reasons, people may be led to believe that they can legitimately ask for death or obtain it for others. Although in these cases the guilt of the individual may be reduced or completely absent, nevertheless the error of judgment into which the conscience falls, perhaps in good faith, does not change the nature of this act of killing, which will always be in itself something to be rejected. The pleas of gravely ill people who sometimes ask for death are not to be understood as implying a true desire for euthanasia; in fact, it is almost always a case of an anguished plea for help and love. What a sick person needs, besides medical care, is love, the human and supernatural warmth with which the sick person can and ought to be surrounded by all those close to him or her, parents and children, doctors and nurses.

III. THE MEANING OF SUFFERING FOR CHRISTIANS
AND THE USE OF PAINKILLERS

Death does not always come in dramatic circumstances after barely tolerable sufferings. Nor do we have to think only of extreme cases. Numerous testimonies which confirm one another lead one to the conclusion that nature itself has made provision to render more bearable at the moment of death separations that would be terribly painful to a person in full health. Hence it is that a prolonged illness, advanced old age, or a state of loneliness or neglect can bring about psychological conditions that facilitate the acceptance of death.

Nevertheless the fact remains that death, often preceded or accompanied by severe and prolonged suffering, is something which naturally causes people anguish.

Physical suffering is certainly an unavoidable element of the human condition; on the biological level, it constitutes a warning of which no one denies the usefulness; but, since it affects the human psychological makeup, it often exceeds its own biological usefulness and so can become so severe as to cause the desire to remove it at any cost.

According to Christian teaching, however, suffering, especially suffering during the least moments of life, has a special place in God's saving plan; it is in fact a sharing in Christ's passion and a union with the redeeming sacrifice which He offered in obedience to the Father's will. Therefore, one must not be surprised if some Christians prefer to moderate their use of painkillers, in order to accept voluntarily at least a part of their sufferings of Christ crucified (cf. Mt. 27: 34). Nevertheless it would be imprudent to impose a heroic way of acting as a general rule. On the contrary, human and Christian prudence suggest for the majority of sick people the use of medicines capable of alleviating or suppressing pain, even though these may cause as a secondary effect semiconsciousness and reduced lucidity. As for those who are not in a state to express themselves, one can reasonably presume that they wish to take these painkillers, and have them administered according to the doctor's advice.

But the intensive use of painkillers is not without difficulties, because the phenomenon of habituation generally makes it necessary to increase their dosage in order to maintain their efficacy. At this point it is fitting to recall a declaration by Pius XII, which retains its full force; in answer to a group of doctors who had put the question: "Is the suppression of pain and consciousness by the use of narcotics...permitted by religion and morality to the doctor and the patient (even at the approach of death and if one foresees that the use of narcotics will shorten life)?" the Pope said: "If no other means exist, and if, in the given circumstances, this does not prevent the carrying out of other religious and moral duties: Yes."[5] In this case, of course, death is in no way intended or sought, even if the risk of it is reasonably taken; the intention is simply to relieve pain effectively, using for this purpose painkillers available to medicine.

However, painkillers that cause unconsciousness need special consideration. For a person not only has to be able to satisfy his or her moral duties and family obligations; he or she also has to prepare himself or herself with full consciousness for meeting Christ. Thus Pius XII warns: "It is not right to deprive the dying person of consciousness without a serious reason."[6]

IV. DUE PROPORTION IN THE USE OF REMEDIES

Today it is very important to protect, at the moment of death, both the dignity of the human person and the Christian concept of life, against a technological attitude that threatens to become an abuse. Thus some people speak of a "right to die," which is an expression that does not mean the right to procure death either by one's own hand or by means of someone else, as one pleases, but rather the right to die peacefully with human and Christian dignity. From this point of view, the use of therapeutic means can sometimes pose problems.

In numerous cases, the complexity of the situation can be such as to cause doubts about the way ethical principles should be applied. In the final analysis, it pertains to the conscience either of the sick person, or of those qualified to speak in the sick person's name, or of the doctors, to decide, in the light of moral obligations and of the various aspects of the case.

Everyone has the duty to care for his or her own health or to seek such care from others. Those whose task it is to care for the sick must do so conscientiously and administer the remedies that seem necessary or useful.

However, it is necessary in all circumstances to have recourse to all possible remedies?

In the past, moralists replied that one is never obliged to use "extraordinary" means. This reply, which as a principle still holds good, is perhaps less clear today, by reason of the imprecision of the term and the rapid progress made in the treatment of sickness. Thus some people prefer to speak of "proportionate" and "disproportionate" means. In any case, it will be possible to make a correct judgment as to the means by studying the type of treatment to be used, its degree of complexity or risk, its cost and the possibilities of using it, and comparing these elements with the result that can be expected, taking into account the state of the sick person and his or her physical and moral resources.

In order to facilitate the application of these general principles, the following clarifications can be added:

– If there are no other sufficient remedies, it is permitted, with the patient's consent, to have recourse to the means provided by the most advanced medical techniques, even if these means are still at the experimental stage and are not without a certain risk. By accepting them, the patient can even show generosity in the service of humanity.

– It is also permitted, with the patient's consent, to interrupt these means, where the results fall short of expectations. But for such a decision to be made, account will have to be taken of the reasonable wishes of the patient and the patient's family, as also of the advice of the doctors who are specially competent in the matter. The latter may in particular

judge that the investment in instruments and personnel is disproportionate to the results foreseen; they may also judge that the techniques
applied impose on the patient strain or suffering out of proportion with
the benefits which he or she may gain from such techniques.
- It is also permissible to make do with the normal means that medicine
can offer. Therefore one cannot impose on anyone the obligation to
have recourse to a technique which is already in use but which carries
a risk or is burdensome. Such a refusal is not the equivalent of suicide;
on the contrary, it should be considered as an acceptance of the human
condition, or a wish to avoid the application of a medical procedure
disproportionate to the results that can be expected, or a desire not to
impose excessive expense on the family or the community.
- When inevitable death is imminent in spite of the means used, it is
permitted in conscience to take the decision to refuse forms of
treatment that would only secure a precarious and burdensome
prolongation of life, so long as the normal care due to the sick person
in similar cases is not interrupted. In such circumstances the doctor has
no reason to reproach himself with failing to help the person in danger.

CONCLUSION

The norms contained in the present Declaration are inspired by a
profound desire to serve people in accordance with the plan of the
Creator. Life is a gift of God, and on the other hand death is unavoidable;
it is necessary, therefore, that we, without in any way hastening the hour
of death, should be able to accept it with full responsibility and dignity. It
is true that death marks the end of our earthly existence, but at the same
time it opens the door to immortal life. Therefore, all must prepare
themselves for this event in the light of human values, and Christians
even more so in the light of faith.

As for those who work in the medical profession, they ought to neglect
no means of making all their skill available to the sick and the dying; but
they should also remember how much more necessary it is to provide
them with the comfort of boundless kindness and heartfelt charity. Such
service to people is also service to Christ the Lord, who said: "As you did
it to one of the least of these my brethren, you did it to me" (Mt. 25: 40).

At the audience granted to the undersigned Prefect, His Holiness Pope
John Paul II approved this Declaration, adopted at the ordinary meeting
of the Sacred Congregation for the Doctrine of the Faith, and ordered its

publication.

Rome, the Sacred Congregation for the Doctrine of the Faith, May 5, 1980.

Franco Cardinal Seper
Prefect
+ Jerome Hamer, O. P.
Tit. Archbishop of Lorium
Secretary

NOTES

1. *Declaration on Procured Abortion*, November 18, 1974: AAS 66 (1974), pp. 730–747.
2. Pius XII, *Address to those attending the Congress of the International Union of Catholic Women's Leagues*, September 11, 1947: AAS 39 (1947), p. 483; *Address to the Italian Catholic Union of Midwives*, October 29, 1951: AAS 43 (1951), pp. 835–854; *Speech to the members of the International Office of Military Medicine Documentation*, October 19, 1953: AAS 45(1953), pp. 744–754; *Address to those taking part in the IXth Congress of the Italian Anaesthesiological Society*, February 24, 1957: AAS 49 (1957), p. 146; cf. also Address on *"reanimation,"* November 24, 1957: AAS 49 (1957), pp. 1027–1033; Paul VI, *Address to the members of the United Nations Special Committee on Apartheid*, May 22, 1974: AAS 66 (1974), p. 346; John Paul II: *Address to the bishops of the United States of America*, October 5, 1979: AAS 71 (1979), p. 1225.
3. One thinks especially of Recommendation 779 (1976) on the rights of the sick and dying, of the Parliamentary Assembly of the Council of Europe at its XXVIIth Ordinary Session; cf. Sipeca, no. 1, March 1977, pp. 14–15.
4. We leave aside completely the problems of the death penalty and of war, which involve specific considerations that do not concern the present subject.
5. Pius XII, *Address* of February 24, 1957: AAS 49 (1957), p. 147.
6. Pius XII, *ibid*, p. 145; cf. *Address* of September 9, 1958: AAS 50 (1958), p. 694.

Originally Published
United States Catholic Conference
June 26, 1980
Reprinted with Permission

NOTES ON CONTRIBUTORS

Francesc Abel, S. J., M. D., Ph. D., Director, Institut Borja de Bioetica, Llaseres, 30, Barcelona, Spain

Benedict M. Ashley, Ph. D., STM, O. P., John Paul II Institute for Studies on Marriage and Family, Washington, D. C. 20017, U.S.A.

Antonio Autiero, Ph. D., Katholisch-theologische Fakultät, der Universität Münster, Münster, Germany

Diana Bader, O. P., Ph. D., Catholic Health Association, St. Louis, MO, 63134–0889, U.S.A.

Thomas J. Bole, III, Ph. D., University of Oklahoma Health Sciences Center, Oklahoma City, Oklahoma, 73190–3046, U.S.A.

Edwin Cassem, S. J., M. D., Department of Psychiatry, Massachusetts General Hospital, Boston, MA, 02114, U.S.A.

Robert C. Cefalo, M. D., Ph. D., Department of Obstetrics and Gynecology, University of North Carolina, Chapel Hill, NC 27599–7570, U.S.A.

John C. Harvey, M. D., Ph. D., Senior Research Fellow, Kennedy Institute of Ethics, Georgetown University, Washington, D. C. 20057, U.S.A.

Kevin O'Rourke, O. P., JCD, STM, Director, Center for Health Care Ethics, St. Louis University Medical Center, St. Louis, MO 63104, U.S.A.

John Paris, S. J., Ph. D., Department of Theology, Boston College, Chestnut Hill, MA, 02167, U.S.A.

Edmund D. Pellegrino, M. D., Director, Center for the Advanced Study of Ethics, Georgetown University, Washington, D. C., 20057, U.S.A.

Paul Schotsmans, Ph. D., Director, Centrum Voor Bio-Medische Ethiek, Kapucijnenvoer 35, B–3000 Leuven, Belgium

Porter Storey, M. D., Director, The Hospice at Texas Medical Center, Houston, TX, 77021, U.S.A.

Kevin Wm. Wildes, S. J., The Center for Ethics, Medicine, and Public Issues, Baylor College of Medicine, Houston, TX, 77030, U.S.A.

INDEX

K.Wm. Wildes (ed.), Birth, Suffering and Death, 227–234.
© 1992 *Kluwer Academic Publishers. Printed in the Netherlands.*

Philosophy and Medicine

KLUWER ACADEMIC PUBLISHERS – DORDRECHT / BOSTON / LONDON